ART, ANGST, AND TRAUMA

Right Brain Interventions with Developmental Issues

Edited by

DORIS BANOWSKY ARRINGTON

W0007636

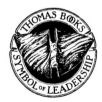

CHARLES C THOMAS • PUBLISHER, LTD.
Springfield • Illinois • U.S.A.

Published and Distributed Throughout the World by

CHARLES C THOMAS • PUBLISHER, LTD.
2600 South First Street
Springfield, Illinois 62704

©2007 by CHARLES C THOMAS • PUBLISHER, LTD.

ISBN 978-0-398-07732-7 (hard)
ISBN 978-0-398-07733-4 (paper)

Library of Congress Catalog Card Number: 2006048897

With THOMAS BOOKS *careful attention is given to all details of manufacturing
and design. It is the Publisher's desire to present books that are satisfactory as to their
physical qualities and artistic possibilities and appropriate for their particular use.*
THOMAS BOOKS *will be true to those laws of quality that assure a good name
and good will.*

Printed in the United States of America
SR-R-3

Library of Congress Cataloging-in-Publication Data

Art, angst, and trauma : right brain intervention with developmental issues / edited by Doris
    Banowsky Arrington.
        p. cm.
    Includes bibliographical references
    ISBN-13: 978-0-398-07732-7
    ISBN-10: 0-398-07732-0
    ISBN-13: 978-0-398-07733-4 (pbk.)
    ISBN-10: 0-398-07733-9 (pbk.)
        1. Brain damage--Treatment. 2. Art therapy. 3. Trauma--Treatment. 4 Brain--Localization
of functions. I. Arrington, Doris Banowsky.

RC387.5.A7834 2007
616.89'1656--dc22

                                                                                2006048897

Dedicated to Christopher William Arrington
1980–2006

My son, Chris, included this commentary in a bulletin he writes each month for staff and faculty in his school district where he is employed as a school psychologist. It is his reflection on the death of my grandson and his nephew.

Chris

I have to believe that events happen in our lives for a reason. And, I have to believe that we are supposed to learn life lessons from those events. Along with my Christian faith, these life lessons give me hope. However, as these events unfold, I am not in the best frame of mind to want to learn a lesson. And sadly, the lessons we're supposed to learn in life often come after the tragic events.

On Monday evening, I watched my oldest brother say goodbye to his 25-year-old son who died two days earlier from a freak motorcycle accident. I am not sure any motorcycle accident is a freak accident. However, it was at that moment that I realized my life lesson in an event so tragic in my family. It was in the Ventura County Morgue, standing with my parents and my two brothers and looking at my nephew that I realized how much my family had taught me about character. The five of us spent 15 short minutes looking at my nephew. We prayed, we cried, we held each other's hands, told stories about my nephew, commented on how beautiful he was, and even made jokes about him. And, then we walked out the doors and watched my brother, his dad, kiss the window goodbye. It was in those short 15 minutes that we shared an entire life. Those same short 15 minutes reaffirmed how important my family is to me and how lucky I am to have a family that taught me the meaning of family. I know I don't thank my parents enough but they did a great job raising three boys and developing character in our lives. I will always have great memories of my nephew but the greatest memory I will have of him is what he taught me about family. I share this part of my life to encourage you to think about what character means to you, to take whatever life gives you and make a better place.

If you died tomorrow, what would people say about you? Would it make you proud of the way you lived and the choices you made? There is an old saying, "If you want to know how to live your life, think about what you would like people to say about you after you die . . . and then live backwards."

It is hard to think now about what will really matter later. But doing so dramatically improves our chances of living a full and meaningful life with few regrets.

Knowing how we want to be remembered allows us to make a sort of strategic plan for our lives. And how much wiser would our choices be if we had the will and discipline to regularly ask ourselves whether all the things we do and say are taking us where we want to be at the end? In a sense, we write our own eulogies by the choices we make every day.

Thanks for letting me share a piece of my life and my thoughts.

His cousin and my granddaughter, Courtney Arrington, age 14, was equally affected by his death. She was one of four 2006 graduation speakers selected by her peers and teachers at Hillview Junior High School. The following is her speech given before graduates and their families at her graduation from the eighth grade.

Courtney

Just because I don't see you doesn't mean I don't love you. These words will forever continue to run through my mind when I think of my Cousin Chris. When he said this to me, I didn't realize it would be one of the last moments in my life I would ever spend with him.

The day was February 4th and the sun was out and shining. I had slept in late because it was the weekend, and around lunch I took a bag of chocolate chips into my parents' bedroom to watch television. The telephone at my house rang and was quickly answered, but I didn't think anything of it.

A few moments later my dad walked into the room where I was watching TV, and pain was spread across his face. He laid down on the bed and put his head on a pillow and closed his eyes. Then after a few seconds, he sat up and looked at me in a way that I will never forget. He looked broken. He said in a crushed voice, "Your cousin Chris has died." Silent tears ran down my father's face as I stared at him in a state of shock. Eventually, hot tears were running down my face as well.

My cousin Chris was a free spirit. He grew up in our family being the fun one that was laid back. Chris, my cousins, and I would stay up until 3 in the morning playing poker and charades and making fun of each other. He was young, 25 years old, and I couldn't understand how his life could be gone. It felt like a piece of my heart was missing, and it still continues to feel like that. After a few moments my dad finally told me that Chris had been in a motorcycle accident. He had hit a fence, and when this happened it broke some of his ribs that then went into and popped his lungs. My heart crumbled into a billion pieces. I had never lost someone that I was so close to or loved so much. Chris was the type of person who could walk into a room and make everyone smile. His life made a huge impact on my life and he will always be remembered.

Through the struggle of trying to understand the loss of Chris in my life, I have found so much comfort in those that I love and those who love me. Before my cousin's death I took love for granted. He made me realize that you have to live every day like it is your last. You have to live your life with a purpose and with love for those you care about.

"Love is patient, love is kind. It does not envy, it does not boast, it is not proud. It is not rude, it is not self-seeking, it is not easily angered, and it keeps no record of wrongs. Love does not delight in evil but rejoices with the truth. It always protects, always trusts, always hopes, and always perseveres. Love never fails." As we leave Hillview Junior High, we need to remember that there are many hellos and goodbyes in life, but the way we live our lives between the hellos and goodbyes is what really counts. We need to remember to love what we have while we have it and not after it's gone. We need to love who we are and what we want to be. Live every day like it is your last, with strong purpose and with love.

CONTRIBUTORS

Editor

Doris Banowsky Arrington, Ed.D., A.T.R.-B.C., licensed clinical psychologist, founding chair of the Graduate Art Therapy Psychology Department at Notre Dame de Namur University, is author of *Home Is Where the Art Is: An Art Therapy Approach to Family Therapy.* Dr. Arrington is active in the American Art Therapy Association (AATA) as a member of the editorial board, committee chair, and former director. The recipient of many awards, she is a Fulbright Senior Specialist and a frequent presenter in the Ukraine, Poland, and China on trauma and art therapy. Her passions include her family, sharing the power of art as healing, and traveling with her husband.

Authors

DeAnn Acton, M.A., A.T.R., M.F.T., art therapist and counselor with School Based Mental Health in San Mateo County, is an adjunct professor at Notre Dame de Namur University. Ms. Acton's passions include her family, painting, performing, and Mexican culture.

Richard Carolan, Ed.D., A.T.R.–B.C., is chair of the Graduate Art Therapy Psychology Department at Notre Dame de Namur University, formerly president of the Art Therapy Credentials Board and associate editor of the *Art Therapy Journal of the AATA.* Dr. Carolan currently mentors 20 research students a year and consults as staff psychologist for a drug and alcohol affiliate of Sutter Health Care System. Dr. Carolan's passions include his family, writing, editing, supervision, and sports.

Araea Rachel Cherry, M.A., A.T.R., M.F.T., certified traumatologist, was the former program director of Children of Domestic Violence in San Mateo County. Cherry trained with the Trauma Response Institute in Morgantown, West Virginia, and with Pia Melody in Arizona. Ahead of her time, Ms. Cherry wrote multiple grants to fund services for children of domestic violence. She was the recipient of the Notre Dame de Namur University Community Service Award. Her passions included her grandsons, drawing, deep conversations, and motorcycling with her life partner. Ms. Cherry died suddenly in August of 2005, leaving a large cadre of saddened family, friends, students, and children at risk.

Angel C. Duncan, M.F.T., A.T.R., is director of *Memories in the Making* and the support group coordinator for the Alzheimer's Association of Santa Clara, San Mateo, and San Francisco counties. Ms. Duncan is also the clinical art therapist at the University of California San Francisco (UCSF) Medical Center, Langley Porter Psychiatric Institute, in both the inpatient and outpatient programs. Her passions include dancing and painting.

Arnell Etherington, Ph.D., M.F.T., A.T.R.-B.C., professor and director of the Marriage Family Therapy Program in the Graduate Art Therapy Psychology Department at Notre Dame de Namur University, was the recipient of the American Art Therapy Association Outstanding Adolescent Clinician Award in 2004 and the Sister Catharine Julie Cunningham Teaching Award in 2006. Dr. Etherington serves on the editorial board for *The Arts in Psychotherapy* and has a private practice in the San Francisco Bay Area. Her passions include painting, travel, and her dog, Teddie.

Linda Gantt, Ph.D., A.T.R.-B.C., H.L.M., is former president of the American Art Therapy Association. She is currently director of the Instinctual Trauma Institute in Morgantown, West Virginia, where she works with traumatized patients. Dr. Gantt has authored and coauthored multiple *AATA Proceedings,* journal articles, and the FEATS: Formal Elements Art Therapy Scale. She and her husband, Dr. Lou Tinnin, present internationally on art therapy and trauma. Dr. Gantt is a Distinguished Scholar at Notre Dame de Namur University. Her passions include her family, writing, working with trauma patients, and fashion design.

David Gussak, Ph.D., A.T.R.-B.C., associate professor and clinical coordinator for the Florida State University Art Therapy Program in the Department of Art Education, is co-editor of the book *Drawing*

Time: Art Therapy in Prisons and Other Correctional Settings. A national and international presenter on art therapy in correctional settings with aggressive and violent clients, Dr. Gussak conducts extensive research about the effectiveness of art therapy in correctional settings. When he is not in his campus office or meeting with clients, he can be found on his bike or kayaking on the river near Tallahassee, where he and his wife, Laurie, have a home.

Roberta Hauser, M.A., A.T.R.-B.C., has over 20 years experience supervising, instructing, and leading creative arts therapy activities for emotionally disturbed children and adolescents. Her passions include her family, crisis intervention, and search and rescue experience in community settings.

Anna Riley Hiscox, M.A., A.T.R.-B.C., M.F.T., co-editor of *Tapestry of Cultural Issues in Art Therapy,* has been active in the AATA as an editor and committee chair. She is an adjunct professor at John F. Kennedy University in Pleasant Hill, California, and a doctoral student at the Institute of Imaginal Studies. Ms. Hiscox has extensive experience in forensic art therapy, domestic violence, and working with severely emotionally disturbed children and adolescents. Her passions include her family, gourd paintings, and printmaking.

Carol Johnson, M.A., A.T.R., M.F.T., is clinical director of the Hospice of the Valley in San Jose, California. Ms. Johnson has been involved with Hospice of the Valley since her practicum days in the late 1980s. In her leisure time, she enjoys caring for her grandson, spending time with her four grown sons, and entertaining family and friends. Her second home is a shared condominium at Lake Tahoe, California, where she hikes in the summer, skis in the winter, and is inspired to paint all year round.

Toni Morley, A.T.R., M.F.T., recently retired from the Alzheimer's Association in Mountain View, California, where she was director of the Memories in the Making Program and facilitated the Early Stage Support groups for Alzheimer's disease. In Spring, 2006, a local media partner awarded Ms. Morley one of the Jefferson Awards for her pioneering work establishing the Memories in the Making program in the Bay Area. Ms. Morley's passions include painting, printmaking, making Polaroid transfers, playing golf, and playing with her three granddaughters.

Sarah Nagle, L.C.S.W., has worked in various aspects of social work for the past 30 years. She gained her M.S.W. from California State University in San Jose and became a licensed clinical social worker in 1999. For the past 12 years, Nagle has dedicated her work to children in foster care. She created and ran the Early Start Program for Aspira Foster Family Agency, which is a program for drug-exposed infants placed in foster care. For the past 6 years she has been director of Daybreak Foster Family Agency in San Jose, California. In addition, she serves as a subject matter expert for the licensing examinations for the Board of Behavioral Sciences. Her passions include her family, friends, and work.

Carolee Stabno, Psy.D., M.F.T., has been a Senior Lecturer for the Art Therapy Psychology Department at Notre Dame de Namur University since receiving her doctorate from Western Graduate School in 1988. Her clinical experiences include private practice, working with children and adolescents (particularly adoptees and children in the foster care system), and chronically mentally ill adults. For over six years she ran a special program for incarcerated males that dealt with substance and physical abuse. Dr. Stabno serves as a subject matter expert for the licensing examinations for the Board of Behavioral Sciences. Her passions include her family, friends, and work.

Lou Tinnin, M.D., former clinical director of the Trauma Recovery Institute in Morgantown, West Virginia, and psychiatrist at Chestnut Ridge Hospital in Morgantown, has been active in the field of art therapy and trauma for over 25 years. A Distinguished Scholar at Notre Dame de Namur University, his passions include fishing, family, and poetry, not necessarily in that order.

JoAnna Wallace, M.A., A.T.R.-B.C., M.F.T., employed by Children's Health Council in Palo Alto, California, is a researcher and author. A doctoral student at Pacific Graduate School, Wallace is interested in neurobiology and art therapy. She has been an adjunct faculty member at Notre Dame de Namur University since 2001. Her passions include surfing, skiing, and hiking.

FOREWORD

In 1976 there was a special art exhibit (In Touch Through Art) organized by Doris Arrington and two other art therapists that focused on the functions of the left and right sides of the brain and the implications for creative activity. The exhibit also featured art with clients with disabilities. The exhibit could best be termed "groundbreaking."

It is synchronistic that in *Art, Angst, and Trauma: Right Hemisphere Interventions with Developmental Issues* we come full circle in terms of understanding how the brain functions and how it is affected by trauma. Of special interest are the two chapters by Arrington on brain development and function. Now of course, there is a lot of neurological and psychological research on the brain, how it develops and how it can be changed by traumatic events. Arrington adds how art therapy can make a major contribution to the healing of trauma because creative activity literally changes the traumatized typography of the brain. She also includes information about the importance of bilateral integration as seen in both Eye Movement Desensitization Reprocessing (EMDR, Parnell, 2006) and art therapy and how this contributes to healing trauma. These chapters are followed by a sequence of chapters devoted to the ways that art therapy facilitates healing of issues throughout the life span.

The volume demonstrates how art therapy can make a major contribution to the treatment of children who are seriously ill, in foster care, physically and emotionally traumatized, as well as deviant and addicted adolescents, young adults, and with the aftermath of a spouse's suicide. The book concludes with a discussion of how art therapy has helped the elderly and their caretakers deal with issues of Alzheimer's and death.

In addition to the broad developmental sweep of the documentation of the success of treatment using art therapy with traumatized clients from early childhood to the elderly, there is a special three-chapter segment on art therapy and a new approach to the treatment of trauma, a reoccurring issue in current society. Gantt and Tinnin have developed a unique way of resolving trauma in which art therapy plays a major role. These professionals termed their approach the Instinctual Trauma Response (ITR). For over a decade, using ITR, they have successfully treated a variety of clients. Images are a crucial component of the ITR. What is especially fascinating is that the client's trauma is resolved without abreaction or re-experiencing the event and without the use of medication (Gantt, 2005; Tinnin, Bills & Gantt, 2002).

Gantt and Tinnin's chapter on the ITR is followed by two chapters by Arrington that illustrate (literally and figuratively) how the ITR works. Among other activities, the client's own graphic narrative of each of the seven steps of the ITR enable verbal narrative and resolution for the client. These cases are from clients Arrington has treated here, and in Eastern Europe. The cases include, the trauma of multiple surgeries, family violence, and witness to death. Of special note is the very detailed and beautifully illustrated case of a wife's trauma in discovering the suicide of her husband.

In addition to the developmental issues threaded through the book there is another "theme" that emerges. This is the multiple rationales for the use of art therapy. In addition to more typical case reports, these rationales are based on neuroscience studies of the brain, the philosophical explanation of how the lack of the ability to visualize can lead the adolescent to addictions. In addition, there is clinical documentation of the successful resolution of different kinds of trauma with a variety of clients, at various stages of development.

Of special note is the chapter on *Adolescents, Identity, Addiction and Image* by Carolan. In the beautiful "flow" of his words, he makes a stunning rationale for the ways art can facilitate identity development. He argues convincingly that art can produce a mind-altering expression without the use of addictive substances.

The chapter, *The Magic Hour: Working with Difficult Children* by Acton and Houser is also noteworthy. I especially liked the charting of their interventions that include: Preparation, Directions, Process Questions, and Goals. This information will be especially helpful to the novice art therapist.

I also congratulate Wallace on her chapter, *Childhood Cancer and Survivorship*. It is well-written and provides excellent and timely information on this subject.

Doris Arrington and her contributors are to be congratulated. This is a book that contains significant *new* material that is a major contribution to the art therapy field.

Frances E. Anderson, Ed.D., A.T.R.-BC, HLM, CPAT

References

Gantt, L. (2005). *Art Therapy and Trauma.* Course materials Florida State University, Tallahassee, Florida.

Parnell, L. (2006, in press). *A therapist's guide to EMDR: Tools and techniques for successful treatment.* New York: W. W. Norton.

Tinnin, L., Bills, L., & Gantt, L. (2002). Short-term treatment of simple and complex PTSD. In: M. Williams & J. Sommer (Eds.), *Simple and complex post-traumatic stress disorder: Strategies for comprehensive treatment in clinical practice* (Chapter 6, pp. 99–118). New York: Haworth Press.

Virshup, E., Eslinger, S. E., & Arrington, D. (1976). *In Touch Through Art,* exhibition catalogue. Fresno Art Center, Fresno, California.

PREFACE

LENA'S FAVORITE KIND OF DAY

The first time I met Lena was at Father's House, a small Christian orphanage outside of Kiev, Ukraine (Arrington & Yorgin, 2001). It was my first short-term medical team trip out of the country and the small voice inside of me wondered why I was there.

After the collapse of communism, unemployment in the former Soviet countries was rampant and continues to be a problem even today. At that time, however, with the welfare system dismantled, parents raised on atheism had no hope and turned to alcohol. Thousands and thousands of children fled abusive parents, unlivable home conditions, and hunger to fend for themselves on the streets of Kiev. To this day, thousands continue to move to the streets. With no papers and no education, the children and the country face an uncertain future. The children find shelter wherever they can, often in steam or sewer systems under the old Soviet-style apartment buildings. They support themselves by begging, stealing, and working as porters or prostitutes.

As Dr. Roman, a gynecologist and obstetrician, was going home late one evening, he met cold and hungry children in the Kiev train station who took him to their shelters. He started that evening taking children from three to fifteen found on the streets and in the train station into his apartment. After his apartment filled with 15, and then 25 children, he found a more amicable setting just outside of Kiev. More and more people heard of this doctor who rescued children living on the streets. We had also heard of Dr. Roman and had been invited to come work with the staff and the children in the orphanage.

The team of American Medical Professionals showed up at the orphanage just as the facility, in a new community, was in the final stage of construction. Dr. Roman, speaking only Russian, met us, led the group in prayer, and then introduced our team to the children. I was surprised when he explained to the team through his interpreter that the children, because of their pain, had been praying for us to come, particularly for a dentist and a psychologist. Yes, their teeth hurt, but due to their traumatic lives of abuse, rejection, isolation, shame, anger, and grief, their hearts hurt as well. Many of the children had never developed trust in or attachment to anyone before moving into Father's House. Indeed, they were having a difficult time, many of them suffering from posttraumatic stress disorder or alexithymia.

While the doctors and nurses worked medically with these children and later with additional children in a state-run orphanage, I spent the week with an interpreter doing art therapy with the same children seen by the doctors. On our first trip we saw over 100 children.

The first thing the team noticed about all of the rosy-cheeked, clean, well-dressed children (in clothes donated from Europe and America) at Father's House was that they rarely smiled. These former street children were without official papers and therefore were unable to attend public schools or receive medical treatment. Many had lived on the streets so long that they had little memory of being a member of a family or an authoritative community that provided them with food, shelter, safety, and moral values.

Hoping to provide a structure of safety, I moved slowly as I assessed the needs of the children. I asked the interpreter to explain to the children how to use the art materials I had brought with me and then I asked them to draw their *favorite kind of day* (Manning, 1987). Lena, a beautiful 12-year-old, curly-headed brunette, was one of those children. While many of the other children talked in Russian among themselves and drew flowers, trees, suns, and people, Lena was one of the sad-faced girls who rarely spoke. She began by drawing a dynamic and violent-looking red gash. Completing the picture, she drew a flower-covered hill around the deep cut. Four sharp, cold, gray mountains grew to meet an encapsulating rainbow and a sky full of dark blue clouds (front cover picture) (Arrington & Yorgin, 2001, pp. 82–83).

Living in California's earthquake country, I saw the red gash as a catastrophe of great magnitude. Cirlot (1962) says an earthquake is "a sudden change in a given process that may be either for the better or for the worse" (p. 93). Rhyne's research (1979) indicates that angular figures in a drawing represent hostility, aggression, and threat.

It was obvious from the art that Lena was expressing thoughts and feelings about her early childhood abandonment. At the time, not even

Dr. Roman knew Lena's past. She had been at the orphanage for fewer than 6 months and as yet did not feel safe. Questioning her in her native language did not help because due to her development, which had been affected by her environment, her language and comprehension skills were limited.

Wanting to know more about the children, I let them lead me, which facilitated my understanding how little the children knew about emotions or how to express them. Dr. Roman invited me to work with the orphanage staff in planning educational games and drama projects around feelings, words, and emotions. Six months later, when I returned to Kiev and to Father's House, I again asked Lena to draw her favorite kind of day. This time, the drawing was more somber and dull, but she repeated her picture of a gash in the earth with many fierce mountains (Arrington & Yorgin, 2001, p. 87).

A year later, Sara, a young Canadian volunteer who spoke Russian, went to live in Father's House with the children. She was able; through her friendship with Lena and through the art directives she had learned as a staff member, to put together the pieces of Lena's life history. Lena, abandoned at about 4 years of age (birthday and age unknown), lived cold and hungry on the streets or in the steam pipes of Kiev with a group of young girls and a large pack of dogs until she was literally picked up around the waist at the age of 11 by one of the orphanage staff and brought to Father's House. While living on the street, the older girls took care of the younger girls, but they often slept together with the dogs for warmth and safety. When Lena, sleeping next to her friend Sara, began to chew on Sara's shoulder, Sara told her she was hurting her and asked her to stop. Lena apologized, explaining that she just wanted Sara to know how much she, Lena, loved her, remarking that snuggling and chewing on them was the way the dogs used to show their affection to the girls who lived with them.

Dr. Roman, never having heard of art therapy, was more than appreciative of it after seeing the first pictures drawn by the children at Father's House. He marveled that a psychologist working with children used art instead of words. He was fascinated to learn how art helped not only the children, but also him and his staff to understand the children's histories and feelings. He was intrigued to find how graphic narratives facilitated the children's use of their verbal skills to talk about their families and life stories.

I have been back to the Ukraine many times, often working with Dr. Roman's sad, unsmiling girls as they come in from the street. Lena taught me the importance of training shelter and orphanage staff in how to use right-hemisphere interventions like art, music, drama, and play to help disadvantaged children make sense of their history and to give them hope for the future.

Doris Banowsky Arrington

References

Arrington, D., & Yorgin, P. (2001). Art therapy as a cross-cultural means to assess psychosocial health in homeless and orphaned children in Kiev. *Art Therapy: Journal of the American Art Therapy Association, 18*(2), 80–89.

Cirlot, J. (1962). *A dictionary of symbols.* New York: Philosophical Library.

Manning, T. (1987). Aggression depicted in abused children's drawings. *The Arts in Psychotherapy, 14*(1), 15–24.

Rhyne, J. (1979). Drawing as personal constructs: A study in visual dynamics. *Dissertation Abstracts International, 79,* 10569.

ACKNOWLEDGMENTS

This book is the evolution of my 35-year-old love affair with art therapy as the treatment modality for mistrust, shame, doubt, guilt, inferiority, identity confusion, isolation and despair and all other life span interruptions. I am truly awed to see neuroscientists begin to document what so many art therapists have known and experienced for a long time, the power of art in healing. This book is about just that, the power of art in healing. The colleagues that have contributed to this book are devoted clinicians who have inspired me with their contributions to bettering the world using art a right hemisphere treatment modality. I am honored by the time and talent they shared with this project and thank them sincerely. I would also like to thank each of my grandchildren, Rett, Ryan, Courtney, Amanda, Connor, Wesley and Haley and their parents for their patience and love during what seemed like an inordinate amount of time. I would like to think my professional family at Notre Dame de Namur University, Richard Carolan, Arnell Etherington, and Carolee Stabno, for their support and help—to my creative student and illustrator Cynthia Gruspy; to my small group members, particularly Carole Courshan for her almost nightly encouragement; to my friends Jan and Jim Rochette who are open to listen; to Frances Anderson, my long-time art therapy buddy who opened my world to writing; to Peter Yorgin, who opened my passion for sharing art therapy with the world; to the clients who have trusted, and risked; to Linda Gantt and Lou Tinnin for their brilliant and generous spirits; to Marsha Calhoun, who likes words; to my editor, Michael Thomas, with his quick answers; and a very special thanks to Bob Arrington, my techie, friend and constant companion who is there with talent and humor at the beginning and at the end. I thank him for a lifetime of help and support of my passion to share art as healing with people around the world.

CONTENTS

ART, ANGST, AND TRAUMA

Chapter 1

LIFE IS BEST LIVED MOVING FORWARD

Doris Banowsky Arrington

Dedicated to Dr. Valerie Appleton, A.T.R.-B.C., M.F.T. (1953–2005),
Dean, Eastern Washington University. Dear friend, the world will
miss your kindness and magic. It was Val who asked, what
could we do today to make life better tomorrow?

Developmental Issues

Developmental theory concerns itself with the phases of human experience and how these phases relate one to another. This book will explore development from the sharp turns, or the traumatic road-blocks that appear along the developmental highway. While interruptions in life are normal, those surfaced in violence can be so devastating and traumatic that they can forever challenge one's movement or direction. This book will document how the graphic and verbal narratives of art interventions effect change in individuals and families, helping them repair and make sense of these powerful and disturbing disruptions. It is my wish that you will find it, as suggested by Fosha (2003), an unfolding conversation from clinical family art therapists informing and transforming neuroscience advances about right-hemisphere interventions. It is my desire that you will be enlightened about the many ways that the right-hemisphere intervention of art therapy touches life, restoring hope and vitality as individuals move forward on life's journey.

As my granddaughter Courtney at age four explained the art piece (Figure 1.1) to her three-year-old cousin, Amanda, "If you are tweated like a princess when you are woodle you gwow up to be a queen"; this is my sincere wish for all young women wherever they are.

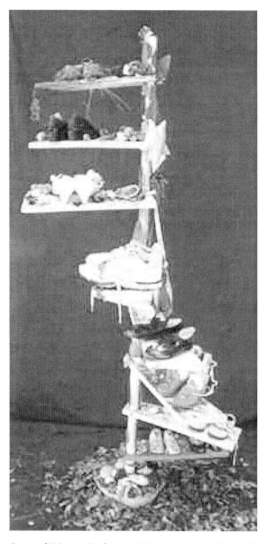

Figure 1.1. *The Eight Steps of Women Sculpture:* Multimedia by Doris Banowsky Arrington.

Erikson's Eight Ages of Humankind[1]

Throughout history, human development has depended on supportive and interactive physical, cognitive, affective, social, and spiritual domains within humanity's only container, the body/mind, to move a human through what Erikson (1963) describes as the Eight Ages of

---

1. In this book, the genders of he and she will be interchangeable.

Mankind. These ages in normal development, with some variations in culture, are consistent across the developmental clock. They begin with the infant and the primary caregiver in the developmental models of Freud's id, Erikson's trust or mistrust, Mahler's object relations, Jung's childhood, and Piaget's sensory motor stage. Erikson (1963) notes that the "strength acquired at any stage is tested by the necessity to transcend it in such a way that the individual can take chances in the next stage with what was most vulnerably precious in the previous one" (p. 263).

Experience dependent, an infant's (0–1 year of age) first goal is to develop trust in his world through a secure attachment with his primary caregiver. A thoughtful and organized beginning of life allows this precious and unique human to develop ease in living, eating, sleeping, and eliminating so that he grows in hope of reaching his maximum complexity physically, cognitively, and affectively (Erikson, 1963; Siegel, 1999).

The inquisitive toddler (2–3 years of age), in Erikson's autonomy stage, begins his journey of independence with the will to make it on his own. He wills to learn, to know, and to hold on or to let go of mother, chairs, toys, and bowel movements. In order to avoid doubt or shame, the toddler learns the social skills of self-control through observation and sensing, motivated by emotions, senses, and acceptance of law and order as perceived by the child's primary caregivers, his parents. Equally important is the climate of the child's living environment. Lewis, Osofsky, and Moore tell us that "clinical studies of children living in areas with high rates of violence report that simply witnessing violence or having knowledge of a violent event can have negative implications" for a child's psychosocial development" (1997, p. 278).

Our child, now 4 years old, is a preschooler. With hope, she moves into Erikson's initiative stage. She learns how to comply in her home, and she knows she has choices. She feels like a big kid but still needs those primary caregivers to recognize her newly-acquired abilities. "Look at me," she yells on the playground. "Look at me." When she is recognized and accepted, she establishes her personhood. Her right-hemisphere experiences of feelings and senses (implicit memory) expand bilaterally through the corpus callosum to the left hemisphere, where they provide structure for explicit memory. Influenced by a sense of time and autobiographical information, they set the stage for the child's motivation of initiative or guilt.

Latency, Erikson's next stage (6–11 years of age) encourages industry. It is a time of "producing things" with skill, domains, ideas, objects, and thoughts while learning to interact in a world with people both inside and outside the family (Erikson, 1963, p. 259). If the child is unable to meet his own demands or those of significant others, inferiority will reign, making life difficult for him and those close to him in his next stage, youth.

Youth (12–19 years of age) appears on the horizon. Childhood is over. Carolan (personal communication, June, 2006) notes that youth or adolescence has long been theorized as a time of crisis in identity development. It is a time in the individual's life where the angst of human experience comes to the foreground. Adolescents, Carolan continues, change in every aspect of their being. Over the course of puberty, testosterone levels increase 18-fold for boys and estrogen levels increase eight-fold in girls. As a result of brain development, adolescent information processing actually changes, moving adolescents into the "formal operations stage" where they are able to reason logically about abstract concepts and develop the capacity for deductive reasoning (Piaget & Inhelder, 1969). They may grow 3 to 8 inches a year for several years, reacting and adjusting to changes in shape and proportion of hands, feet, and bodies. They often have a heightened sense of sensation seeking, finding this in peer rather than family relationships. Even their moral development is thought to go through major changes. From Freud's perspective (as cited in Bee & Boyd, 2003), the move through the latency stage and into the genital stage activates libidinal energy, which must be appropriately channeled. Identity formed from past experiences helps shape who the adolescent is, but current interests and behaviors redefine it. All of this manifests in their lives what Erikson (1963) calls an identity crisis, in which the individual's psychological process of identity development exists in a moratorium between childhood and adulthood (Bee & Boyd, 2003). This moratorium can stall the adolescent's need for identity and commitment to a belief, a person, or a purpose. Environmental risk and protective factors, important in this stage, influence adolescent development whether it be identity or identity crises.

The young adult, now in his twenties and thirties, builds on interests developed in adolescence or searches for new ones. He looks for commitment and a partner who will share his work, his dreams, and his ultimate concerns. Somewhere between 20 and retirement, that large span of adulthood, his horizons expand beyond his personal journey. He looks outside of himself for purpose, and forms partnerships with the desire to eventually give back and guide the next generation. Generativity, an essential element in the psychosexual and psychosocial model, has a giving-back-agenda. The adult assumes responsibility and purpose, "gardening in the great forests of the world" (Arrington, 1985), caring for his community and serving others, family, or humanity. Without landscape interests broader than self, one is limited and isolated.

Old age comes quickly. The senior, in his sixties or seventies, is healthier today than he was in the past. If, in each stage of life, he has met developmental goals of trust, autonomy, initiative, industry, identity, intimacy, and generativity, he will come to this final stage with wisdom, having lived uniquely and yet interrelated to all other humans. His travels will have taken him far, teaching him how to let go of his need for control and to trust the journey. If he has not been able to integrate life's developmental goals, life's ending will be one of loss, sadness, and despair.

Finally, the frail elderly, ages 60 to 100 years old, represents a group in Western society that is living longer, healthier lives with a variety of opportunities. The emotional state in these later years will depend not only on health but also on how well the individual has traveled in the earlier stages of life and met the challenges of each.

The ages mentioned above are not rigid because humans are dynamic. Some love and work successfully from early childhood to frail elderhood, others love and work sporadically, and still others never find success in either category. Life, however, is more than a theoretical approach. On a daily basis, all humans meet life and its large and small interruptions. Those interruptions, good or ill, stop us, delay us, or lead us into new internal views. Life, all life, includes the interruptions, the detours, the roadblocks and the developmental disasters that happen to the soul, the intellect, and the mind of individuals and families along life's journey. Life is actually filled with a myriad of experiences and emotions—joy, acceptance, fear, surprise, sadness, disgust, anger, and anticipation—with all of their direct and alternative responses. It is also filled with death and for far too many people, violence. Death is a natural part of life: death of experiences, death of relationships, and finally death, the end of life itself. Not everyone, on the other hand, experiences violence. Therefore, when violence is in the home or the neighborhood, like fog on the road, it blankets the environment, impacting children's development. According to Lewis et al. (1997, p. 279), it erodes their "sense of personal safety and security," disrupting their "lifestyle and the major ages of socialization." Violence "generalizes emotional distress." It depersonalizes the people involved in it or witnessing it, and at the same time it "diminishes their future orientation." We, as professional clinicians, ask how do we assist others in their struggles through life's difficult roads and highways?

Conclusion

In the months since I started collaborating on this book, my life, in the metaphor of the road, has been in almost constant interruption by roadblocks, washouts, or repair. It has been clouded over with constant change. It seems that I *learn by going where I have to go* (Roethke, 1953). It began with my husband of many years painfully and slowly recovering from a year of ill health and difficult treatment. In the fall, my former student, office partner, friend, and co-author of several chapters in this book, Rachel, died suddenly, with conversations unfinished, notes untitled, and art unidentified. This was followed by the long and painful December death of Valerie, one of my first and most beloved students and friends. In February the life of my grandson, a beautiful 25-year-old, was cut short by a motorcycle accident. His death broke all of our hearts, as you can tell by the dedications from his uncle and cousin. This week, a friend's 17-year-old daughter, volunteering in a beauty salon providing services for marginalized women, was hit in the spine by a bullet when one of the women dropped her bag and her loaded pistol went off accidentally. The spinal cord of the teenager was severed and the owner of the gun, a young mother with a 2-year-old and a 3-year-old, went to jail. My husband's 94-year-old mother is slowly slipping into the next world and I have just retired from a job I have loved for 30 years. However, as I write about the death of one experience, the roundabout on the road brings me to new opportunities on many different fronts.

I include the above events because they are developmental parts of life, my life. They are the landscapes that identify my life journey as unique. They are the events that challenge and put emotion and color into all I do. They flesh out my skeleton of living. They transform my soul.

Each one of us faces life, death, and development with events, occurrences, and conditions specific to us. Each of us has a life chock full of challenges that make it up: a child getting cancer, or one with a learning disability; losing a job; returning to school; having too many pregnancies, or not enough; getting a boob job, a knee job, a triple bypass; a family member dying naturally. When a child is taken from a neglectful or an abusive parent, when a teenager becomes addicted to alcohol or drugs, when fights in a marriage turn to battering, or when a teenager is paralyzed by a stray bullet when she is just volunteering for a senior project, violence has intervened. Confusion and angst erode our sense of security. Sadness is overwhelming. However stressful or traumatic our experiences may be, they are the blood, tissue, and muscles of life.

As you read this book, I encourage you to look at what you consider roadblocks or interruptions in your own life. Someone once said life is not for the weak of heart. Being the elder that I am, I believe that life is learning to trust, to risk, and to grow with the roadblocks and to seek professional help for the horrific experiences that slow down or halt what we consider our life movement. This book addresses some of those experiences, interventions, and the people affected. It addresses right-hemisphere interventions, art as treatment, a true passion of the people who contributed to this book. Art therapy helps people "comprehend frightening and confusing traumatic experiences" and move forward on their own unique developmental highways (Lewis et al., 1997, p. 280).

References

Arrington, D. (1985). *Gardening in the great forest: Life review of the stages of development through art therapy.* Burlingame, CA: Abbeygate Press.

Bee, H., & Boyd, D. (2003). *Lifespan development* (3rd ed.). Boston: Allyn and Bacon.

Erikson, E. (1963). *Childhood and society* (2nd ed.). New York: W. W. Norton

Fosha, D. (2003). Dyadic regulation and experiential work with emotion and relatedness in trauma and disorganized attachment. In M. Solomon & D. Siegel (Eds.)., *Healing trauma: Attachment, mind, body and brain* (pp. 221–281). New York: W. W. Norton.

Lewis, M., Osofsky, J., & Moore, M. S. (1997). Violent cities, violent streets. Children draw their neighborhoods. In J. Osofsky (Ed.), *Children in a violent society* (pp. 277–299). New York: Guilford Press.

Piaget, J., & Inhelder, B. (1969). *The psychology of the child* (H. Weaver, Trans.). New York: Basic Books.

Roethke, T. (1953). *The Waking. Poems 1933–1953.* Garden City, NY: Doubleday.

Seigel, D. (1999). *The developing mind: Toward a neurobiology of interpersonal experience.* New York: Guilford Press.

Chapter 2

THE MANY WAYS OF KNOWING

Doris Banowsky Arrington

Dedicated to Araea Rachel Cherry, my student, friend, office partner, and co-author, who died last August as we were beginning to write this chapter. The angels must have needed your insight and generous spirit.

Introduction

> Everything starts and ends in your mind. How your mind works determines how happy you are, how successful you feel, how much time you perceive that you have in life and how well you interact with other people. The patterns of your mind encourage you toward success or drive you to failure. (Amen, 1998, p. 90)

This chapter briefly explores the functions and purposes of the brain: its anatomy, its structures, its way of knowing, and how these foundational structures of thinking and feeling are interrelated. It will look at how these structures communicate perceived reality and self-awareness both visually and verbally in healthy and adverse circumstances.

Many people in the Western world believe that intellect is the only way of knowing. Humans, however, have two minds, one that thinks and one that feels. They actually have many ways of knowing. The appropriateness and expression of thinking, feeling, and knowing are shaped in a "childhood and adolescent window of opportunity" (Goleman, 1995, p. 8). Today, this information is supported by research in the neurosciences (Felitti, 2004; Solomon & Siegel, 2003).

The notion of the mind comes from the word *psyche,* defined by *Webster's New World Dictionary* (Neufeldt & Guralnik, 1966) as soul, intellect, or mind. In brief, the soul is the seat and vitality of real life. The intellect is the capacity for logic and knowing and the mind is the capacity for memory, intention, purpose, choice, and wish. Kaplan (2000) refers to the mind as conscious and unconscious streams of coded representations. These "representations correspond to perceptions and the memory and manipulation of perceptions" (p. 38).

The Developing Mind

At birth, babies already have approximately 100 million neurons. These units make up the infant's nervous system, communicating within and between the undeveloped brain as well as with the rest of the body. These patterns, or flows of energy and information, activate the brain. Prior to two years of age, senses, feelings, and undated and nonautobiographical events form implicit memories. These neurons, and possibly even some before birth, adapt their trillion of synapse connections from one to another. Dendrites attract incoming information to the cell nucleus, and axons conduct information away (Carter, 1998, p. 14; Lambert, Bramwell, & Lawther, 1982).

The human brain, experience-dependent, alters and is altered by other minds (Siegel, 2003). It regulates internal patterns or flows of energy and information, while interacting and exchanging this flow with the external world. It is driven, not by central organization, but by collaborative communication in such areas as needs, senses, and emotions in a system of super systems with their own terms and language.

Piaget, ahead of his time, observed that an infant's brain begins development with a series of fleeting pictures (Elkind, 1985). As the developing child, through assimilation and accommodation, progressively brings patterns of energy and information together with those fleeting pictures, he constructs the schema of permanent objects. He develops brain connections that create an emerging sense of self in a mind consisting of both cognitive and emotional intelligence (Siegel, 1999, 2003). Sensory images, says Lusebrink (1990), are the bridge for integrating information in the mind with physiological changes in the body.

In the late 1920s, while researching the development of intelligence in infancy and early childhood, Piaget found that intelligence develops in a series of age-related stages that cannot be hurried. Today, a major goal of psychoneurology is to discern how humans think and how early brain patterns and stages drive individuals toward "maximal complexity" with structures that equip one for developmental success or restrict structures that will lead to developmental failure (Seigel, 2003). The major goal of psychotherapy is to use that information in treating the pathology of patients to determine how and why humans think effectively. In treating patients, we know that self-narratives that reflect success are clear, understandable, and coherent, whereas those that are confused and incoherent do not.

Brief Synopsis of Brain Purpose, Structure, and Function. (For those less interested in the biology and functions of the brain you may want to move on to the next section called The Developing Brain.)

The **purpose** of the brain is goal-directed behavior. The brain is the coordinator of emotional and mental activity. The **function** of the brain is information processing through alertness, action, and activity. The five senses–taste, touch, hearing, smelling, and seeing–feed information to the **brain stem** that weaves this information together before directing it to the rest of the body, where it regulates or deregulates breathing, heart rhythm, and blood pressure.

Each brain module, except for the pineal gland, is duplicated in both the right and the left hemisphere. Both hemispheres of the cerebrum, connected by the 20 million-fiber network of the corpus callosum, are divided into four lobes with specific but not necessarily singular purposes (Carter, 1998). The **frontal lobe** develops gradually and is believed to integrate, among other things, language, conceptualizing, planning, and emotional reactions. The **parietal lobe** is believed to be involved with movement, eye-hand orientation and coordination, body image, calculations, and certain types of recognition. The **occipital lobe** is concerned with visual processing and recognition. The **temporal lobe** includes centers for sound, speech, some memory, and organization. The **cerebellum** is involved with movement and balance. The **pons** controls breathing and heartbeat. The **frontal (neo) cortex** is the seat of thought, strategizing, and long-range planning. It integrates art and culture, and right-hemisphere mother-child bonding. The **limbic system** of the brain is the emotional generator, integrating learning and memory and arousing or tempering feelings that range from anger to love. The **amygdala** is the brain's alarm clock for fear and perceived danger. The **meninges,** the protective membranes that cover the brain, are involved with long-term memory, as is the **hippocampus.** The **thalamus** works as a relay system, directing incoming information to appropriate parts of the brain and the body. Finally, the **hypothalamus** keeps the body adjusted to the environment (Carter, 1998; Damasio, 1994). Carter (1998) describes the brain as the "size of a cocoanut, shaped like a walnut; the color of liver and the consistency of cold butter" (p. 15).

Like lights during the Christmas season, one neighbor brain cell after another, virtually instantaneously, in orchestrated webs of connections, fires transmitting information and impulses through the release of **hormones** and other **neurotransmitters** (Damasio, 1994).

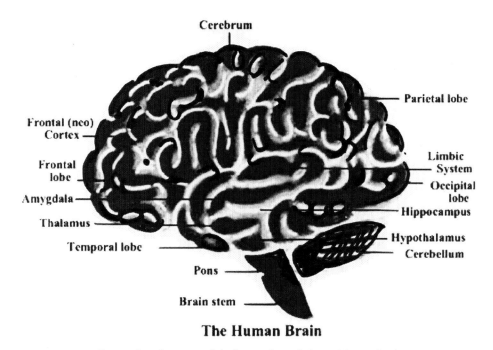

Figure 2.1. *Structure of the human brain* (adapted by author).

The most important neurotransmitters, chemicals that when released into spaces between fired-up cells produce simultaneous activity, are dopamine, acetylcholine (ACTH), serotonin, noradrenaline, glutamate, and endorphine (Carter, 1998, p. 29). Neuroscientists believe that it is the location of these firings that determines the nature of the emerging mental processes. How essential are those early fleeting images to brain development? What should psychotherapists in general and creative art psychotherapists specifically know about this process?

The Developing Brain Structure

According to Klorer, "Neuralplasticity . . . is the brain's ability to change its structure in response to environmental stimuli" (2005, p. 214). For example, connections, sparse at birth, constantly seek new stimuli. One neuron may relate to 10,000 other neurons, but rarely do the neurons communicate with any that are not close by or in a similar system. With both highly charged emotional experiences (stress) and consistent activation (routine), neuropathways are stimulated and brain structure changes. When states of being like love, trust, fear, or aggression are reinforced, pathways develop into patterns or traits of behavior. As these states become traits, they are passed on to the next generation.

A safe and nurturing environment provides the opportunity for the infant (0–2 years old) and then the young child (3–5 years old) to develop a state of trust, i.e., choosing close proximity to a caregiver, feeling secure and safe enough to be willing to leave the caregiver and explore the universe. Unfortunately, the child who feels unsure and threatened will limit exploring without understanding why. This is important in brain development because around the age of 6, the brain, having reached its maximum neural density, will begin to decrease that neural density as neuron cells are pruned through redirection or lack of use.

An excess or depletion of neurotransmitters, the brain's chemical bridges, also changes the brain's behavior patterns, structure, and physical processes (LeDoux, 1996). For example, increased levels of serotonin cause fusion, agitation, and motor abnormalities. Decreased levels of serotonin cause depression (Carter, 1998). Klorer (2005) believes a secure environment, with limited stress, is essential to maintaining healthy consistency in neurotransmitters.

Example: Holly and Ryan. Holly, age 22 months, and her brother, Ryan, just turning 4, give us an example. Both are good, sweet kids. Dad's job requires him to go to work early. This leaves Mom, depressed and on tranquilizers, asleep, so the kids have learned to fix cereal and watch cartoons. They know to be quiet and help Mom during the day when she is cranky. When Mom takes her 4 p.m. nap, the kids eat cookies, pick their TV shows, and wait until Daddy comes home to fix dinner. What are the kids learning about trust? Will one or both grow up to be like mother, depressed and needy?

Trust patterns learned during the attachment phase (ages 0–5) build brain structures that assist in the brain's ability to be flexible, to go with the flow, to trust the process, and to see options. Patterns and structures of mistrust in this area, also learned during the attachment phase, can lead to distractibility, impulsiveness, procrastination, and poor decision-making abilities. These limited responses preclude attachment patterns of security, self-soothing, and being in control, instead encouraging patterns that reflect worry, stubbornness, obsessive-compulsiveness, oppositional behaviors, and addictions. "A growing body of studies indicates that traumatic childhood experiences provide the context for the roots of adult violence" (Schore, 2003, p. 108).

Emotions

"Various researchers claim to have identified the primary emotions, usually as disgust, fear, anger and parental love. These are the responses that seem to be displayed by nearly all living things of any complexity" (Carter, 1998, p. 83). The emotion of anger results in wanting to fight with the blood flowing to the arms. The emotion of fear, when one wants to flee, sends the blood flowing to the larger skeletal muscles, the legs. Overwhelming or constant fear results in feeling numb, unable to move, as if frozen. When one feels sadness, there is a drop in energy. When one is surprised, the retina widens to look closer. Disgust arises when one is left with an offensive taste or smell. Love is associated with feelings of calm and contentment. And happiness is an emotion that inhibits negative energy. Complex emotions are mixtures of primary emotions that mixed with cognitive processing, result in physical responses such as guilt, shakes, tingles, butterflies, gutaches, breathlessness, muscle tension, warmth, and more.

Developing Emotional Structure

If we did not have feelings and emotions that reflected our likes and desires, making choices, maintaining relationships, and calculating plans would be ineffective, if not impossible.

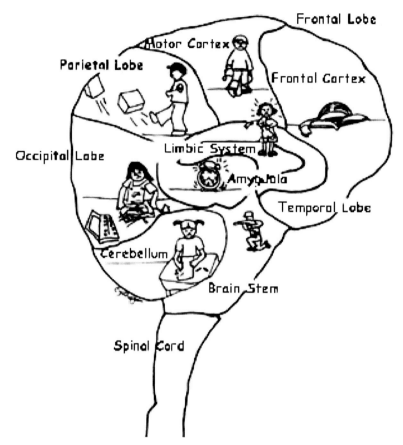

Figure 2.2. *An artist's illustration of the interior working of a brain belonging to a person who is insecurely attached to a primary caregiver.* (C. Gruspy, artist)

Basic emotions are not just feelings; each emotion is a feeling and a survival action or response. For example, I feel afraid **and** I fight, run, or freeze. I feel angry **and** I fight or walk away. I feel hungry **and** I find food to eat (LeDoux, 1996). During the past six years, I have trained over 200 staff in the Ukraine who work with street children and I have observed, assessed, and treated over 300 street kids living in orphan-ages or government shelters. The art of many of these rejected and abused children reflects their self-identity, not as humans with feelings, but as strange and confused-looking monsters. Without positive adult

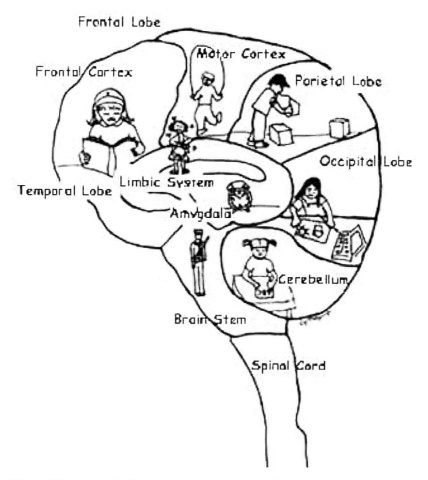

Figure 2.3. *An artist's illustration of the interior of a brain belonging to a person who is securely attached to a primary caregiver.* (C. Gruspy, artist)

interactions like those that occur during the attachment phase, street children around the world grow up to become the monsters they project. If no one has helped them see themselves as human beings with feelings of love and empathy, why would we assume that they would be able to be empathic or compassionate to other humans they meet randomly on the street?

The following drawings of "a person" are by two teenage boys who live on the streets in Eastern Europe. One was charged with assault and the other was a perpetrator of sexual crimes.

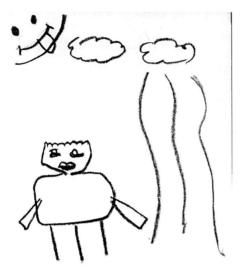
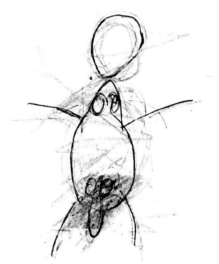

Figure 2.4. *Draw a person.*   Figure 2.5. *Draw a person.*

Bilateral Integration

The right hemisphere of the brain, known for being more dominant in the first three years of life, is the base for implicit information as in attachment and building trust in a child. Beyond cortical energy and nonverbal information, the right hemisphere absorbs emotions, facial expressions, tones, and ways to soothe the inner world of the self. For the psychotherapist wanting to help clients develop these positive patterns, Siegel's (2003) suggestion that the right hemisphere mediates "the retrieval of autobiographical memory" (p. 15) is both noteworthy and instructive. For example, nonverbal therapeutic retrieval processes follow right-hemisphere sensory patterns. These patterns respond to, crawling, alternately tapping hands or shoulders, marching, eye movement, and electronic stimulation as seen in EMDR (Parnell, 2006). They also respond to drawing, coloring or painting, as well as images that have been previously selected in order to describe or represent feelings and experiences (DeLue, 1994). Graphic art, specifically, is a way nonverbal memories communicate nonverbally. Educational psychologist John Allan (1988) tells us that art is a vehicle to the unconscious.

Although the left hemisphere is what has made humanity the outstanding species it is in creating and producing, the right brain is the location for the subjective awareness of primary emotions like attachment, anger, fear, or trust (Carter, 1998). Early childhood facilitates right-hemisphere structure development of human closeness and security from sensory information, fleeting images, and implicit memories. Between the ages of one and two years, when the hippocampus and the prefrontal cortex are established and shaped by attachment processes, explicit autobiographical memory begins to develop, equipping left-hemisphere structures that learn linearly, logistically, and linguistically (Siegel, 2003). The left hemisphere, with these extremely capable qualities, is the designated driver of the child's sense of worth. They influence the child's need to understand and to tell his life story as he learns about the outer world. If there is a blockage, as occurs in people with extreme stress or posttraumatic stress disorder (PTSD) (American Psychological Association, 1994), then the story of the self may be incomplete and incoherent (Siegel, 2003). This does not appear to be the case in the following story recently reported in the local paper. Although Ashley's beginnings were dangerous, she obviously had a secure attachment and found meaning in her life story.

Example: Ashley. Ashley, soon after her birth 18 years ago, was found in a brown paper bag, on the side of a highway by a Highway Patrol officer who had stopped for a brief rest. Recently, she graduated with 285 other members of her high school graduating class. This fall, Ashley will attend an out-of-state university on a scholarship. Although her whole childhood is replete with both miracles and traumas, many people cared for her. Ashley knows her life story and recognizes that she is here for a purpose. She told family and friends attending her high school graduation party, "I'm here to do something with my life, I am not here to sit around and cry and waste my time thinking about what happened to me" (Rubenstein, 2006, p. B3).

The Emotional Brain

"Human emotions are rather like colors: there seems to be a handful of primary ones [anger, anticipation, joy, acceptance, fear, surprise, sadness, disgust] and a wider range of more complex concoctions created by mixing the primary ones together" [rage, vigilance, ecstasy, adulation, terror, amazement, grief, and loathing] (Carter, 1998, p. 82). Emotions do not require consciousness to respond. Instead, emotion, once it has been activated, immediately activates the amygdala that responds with both innate and learned survival responses. Emotional patterns, when mixed unconsciously, can produce highly complicated feelings and responses, sometimes with catastrophic results (Carter, 1998). Positive patterns of attachment, love, trust, and safety permeate the right hemisphere, regulating amygdala influences and producing low levels of cortisol (hormones and neurotransmitters). The amygdala, the specialist for emotional matters, is based on a working memory that begins with the activation of the senses, i.e., hearing, seeing, smelling, tasting, or touching (LeDoux, 1996). The image of the sensory object travels by chemical bridge to the thalamus. When the information is not hyper aroused, it goes from the thalamus to the neocortex and then to the hippocampus, where the image integrates current sensory memory with experience. Depending on whether the sensory object is something pleasant, needed, or threatening, the response from the amygdala will be quite different.

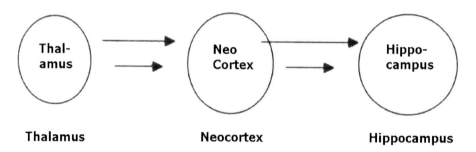

Figure 2.6. *Sensory object chemical bridge.*

Motivated by the senses, hyper-aroused neural energy and information travel differently. They move from the thalamus to the amygdala, the brain's alarm system, that when stressed by anger, fear, and shame, activates the brain with a perception of immediate danger before sending the information to the hypothalamus. The body, alerted by the amygdala and perceiving attack, reacts, etching patterns of excitement and fragmentation into the brain. That energy and information will not go away, but will reappear randomly in the person's thoughts. When allowed to come to closure in the form of a life story that makes sense and can be understood, that energy and information no longer responds to random brain patterns and fragmentations perceived as danger.

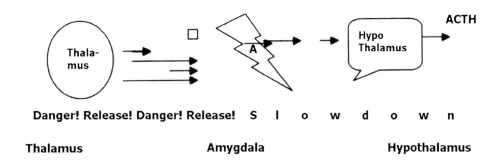

Thalamus   **Amygdala**   **Hypothalamus**

Figure 2.7. *Hyper-aroused chemical bridge.*

These negative patterns inhibit the working memory and the attention of the prefrontal cortex, producing high levels of cortisol. When panic or fear is sustained in the presence of stimuli, cortical chemicals etch the senses of the trauma (panic or fear) into the right hemisphere alarm system. The person, now in a panic, reacts by fighting, fleeing, or freezing, with patterns that affect facial expressions, automatic nervous system changes (anxiety), dendrite shrinkage (memory loss), as well as cortical chemical and hormonal changes (physical shock responses such as palpitations, body weakness, and breathing difficulties), often causing PTSD. One has only to remember the reaction of those in the vicinity of the Twin Towers on September 11 to have a working memory of the human's reaction to fear and danger.

Memory

Memory, the retained knowledge of previous occurrences, fact, thoughts, and feelings, is also a way of knowing. Relevant memory cues are those from the mind and body that signal that the person is in the same emotional state that he or she was in during the original experience. Researchers believe that extensively connected neural pathways, those pathways that have been traveled many times, make retrieval easier and memory more vivid. Limited neural pathway connections, those traveled less frequently, make memory more difficult (Carter, 1998; Damasio, 1994; LeDoux, 1996; Siegel, 2003).

With all that is known about the brain and its functions, there is still much that is unknown. Neuroscientists hesitate about assigning specific tasks to one part of the brain. Seigel (2003), building on this, points out that knowledge is always a construction in process. The brain is not a filing cabinet, a library, or even a computer, with parts that are task specific. It is a complex system with interrelated parts that are dynamic, always adjusting to both inner and outer stimuli. Damasio (1994) explains that "each memory [image] is a newly reconstructed version of the original" but not the original, because the brain, within a window of time, has the means to reconstruct an approximate representation from the firing synapse patterns that have been strengthened through branches of axons and dendrites or weakened because of lack of experience or use (p. 100). The figures below are an artist's depiction of active axons that have been strengthened and inactive axons that have been weakened.

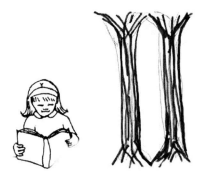

Figure 2.8. *Strengthened:* Artist's depiction of active axons.

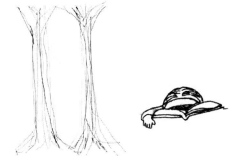

Figure 2.9. *Weakened:* Artist's depiction of inactive axons.

Researchers and therapists are learning that with appropriate therapeutic interventions, those that use bilateral integration of both right and left hemispheres, the severity of most traumatic experiences can be remediated or resolved.

Stress

Stress puts pressure on the mind and body, impacting memory differently than nonstressful events. Modules within the brain's limbic system are capable of learning and remembering highly-charged emotional events, even those experienced during infancy. Throughout life, those cortical modules control appetite, sleep cycles, heart rate, and blood pressure. They modulate libido, process senses, and help people bond. Under stress, the adrenal glands release steroids into the blood, alerting the amygdala, which reacts by signaling its neighbor, the hypothalamus, of danger. The hypothalamus activates processes that release adrenal corticosteriods or ACTH (see Figures 2. 7 and 2.10). ACTH releases stress hormones into the system that slow down or stop brain processes. Restricted and under severe stress, the amygdala signals, "Help! Help! Danger! Release (high cortisol)! Danger! Release (high cortisol)!" while the hippocampus, trying to restore order, signals, "S l o w d o w n, s l o w   d o w n " (LeDoux, 1996, p. 241). When the hippocampus is overworked from trying to slow down and restore order in the body, it causes moodiness, negativity, and finally depression. In addition, as discussed earlier, it will shut down, inhibiting learning and memory and damaging the immune system.

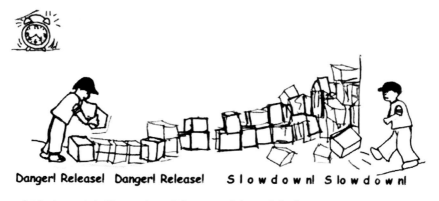

Danger! Release! Danger! Release!   S l o w d o w n!   S l o w d o w n!

Figure 2.10. An artist's illustration of the amygdala and the hippocampus under stress.

Because stress is cumulative and damaging, restricting both the quantity and quality of hormones and neurotransmitters, it reduces the ability to produce new and reconstructive images that become thoughts and later memories (Damasio, 1994). These traumatic images from unresolved trauma may allow implicit memory (emotional) processing but block explicit memory (cognitive) storage (Siegel, 2003), resulting in negative flashbacks, flooded emotions, bad memories, and dreams altering heartbeat, blood pressure, and emotions (Carter, 1998). If an individual has been exposed to extreme trauma, the firing synapse patterns in the right hemisphere will either have been flooded and out of control because of too many traumatic images, as in posttraumatic stress disorder (PTSD), or will shut down from overload (like the hypothalamus), producing no images, as in alexithymia (van der Kolk, McFarlane, & Weisath, 1996).

Adverse Childhood Experiences

The brains of children who experience adverse childhoods are significantly affected throughout their lifetimes (Arrington & Cherry, 2004). Adverse childhood experiences (ACE) are common, destructive, and the most important determinants of the physical and mental health and well-being of adults. Children who suffer relational trauma through neglect, abuse, family loss, community trauma, environmental disasters, or medical invasions risk the over-pruning of cortical neurons. This toxic condition results in the death of those important neuronal pathways within the neo cortex (thinking) and the limbic system (feeling), which are responsible for emotional regulation (Seigel, 1999, p. 85). Overwhelming stress can exacerbate this situation (Shore, 1997), damaging the very soul of a person, the seat of his or her vitality of living, for life. Neurobiological brain structures of children who have experienced these adverse conditions may be so damaged that they cannot be repaired, even with pharmaceuticals, as in the case of severely maltreated children, as well as some chronically ill and mentally ill adults and most felons.

In the mid-1980s, Dr. Robert Anda, of the Centers for Disease Control (CDC), and Dr. Vincent Felitti, of Kaiser Permanente Hospital in San Diego, conducted a study that revealed a powerful relationship between the emotional experiences of children and the physical and mental health of those children after reaching adulthood. The Adverse Childhood Experience Study (ACE Study) examined 17,421 overweight adults with an average age of 57 (Felitti, 2004, p. 1). The project derived from staff observations in an obesity program that there was a high rate of dropouts who surprisingly were losing weight. The connecting feature from the interviews conducted by the researchers was that all of the weight-losing dropouts had experienced sexual abuse predating their weight gain. No previous person or study had made the connection of excess weight being a protective solution to the abuse problem. In the ACE Study, eight categories of household dysfunction were studied. These included the following dysfunctions:

- Recurrent physical and emotional abuse
- A family member who was chronically depressed, suicidal, or mentally ill
- Sexual abuse
- Emotional or physical neglect
- Drug or alcohol abuser in the family
- The mother was treated violently
- An incarcerated household member
- At least one biological parent was lost to the subject during childhood, regardless of the cause

To compare distant childhood experiences, cohorts were studied for five years. An individual exposed to none of the categories had an ACE score of 0. "An individual exposed to any four of the categories had an ACE score of 4" (Felitti, 2004, p. 2). Adult categories of health studied included smoking, chronic obstructive pulmonary disease (COPA), hypertension, diabetes, obesity, substance abuse, and attempted suicide. As ACE scores increased, individuals were found to be more at risk for heart disease, diabetes, obesity, unintended pregnancy, sexually transmitted diseases, fractures, and alcoholism. The study clearly identifies that ACE is common, destructive, and has a lifetime effect. The prevention aspects are positively daunting.

Conclusion

The mind has many ways of knowing and perceiving reality. These include the use of both right and left hemispheres of the brain cognitively and emotionally, through the senses, under stress, and from memory. Siegel and Hartzell (2003) note that experiences or "neural firings turn on the genetic machinery that allows the brain to change its internal connections or memory" (p. 34). The nonverbal right brain, with its implicit memory, is present at birth and continues throughout the life span (p. 23). It creates mental models of generalizations of repeated experiences, like the comforting or lack of comforting experiences of attachment between a child and her caregiver. Although recalled implicit memories do not include awareness of the early experiences, they do reflect them and shape how humans perceive, act, and respond throughout their lives.

Explicit memory, on the other hand, utilizes these fired neuron connections made by implicit memory experiences, encoding their process. Between the ages of one and two, once brain structures are established and shaped by early relational experiences, explicit autobiographical memory begins to develop. As seen in those who have undergone adverse childhood experiences, unhealthy environments thwart the brain's ability to develop successfully, whereas healthy environments promote integrative capacities, enabling children to thrive, to be productive, and to reach their maximum complexity.

References

Allan, J. (1988). *Inscapes of the child's world*. Dallas, TX: Spring.

Amen, D. (1998). *A clinician's guide to understanding and treating ADD: The clinician's tool box*. Fairfield, CA: Mindworks Press.

American Psychiatric Association. (1994). *Diagnostic and Statistical Manual of Mental Disorders* (4th ed.). Washington, DC: American Psychiatric Association.

Arrington, D., & Cherry, R. (2004). Long-term intergenerational affects of violent families: Frozen in fear. In *35th Annual Conference Proceedings of the American Art Therapy Association* (p. 134). San Diego, CA. American Art Therapy Association, Inc.

Carter, R. (1998). *Mapping the mind*. Berkeley, CA: University of California.

Damasio, A. (1994). *Descartes' error: Emotion, reason and the human brain*. New York: Avon.

DeLue, C. (1994). *The physiological effects of children creating mandalas*. Unpublished master's thesis, College of Notre Dame, Belmont, CA.

Elkind, D. (1985). *Piaget's developmental theory: An overview with David Elkind, PhD* [Motion picture]. (Available from Davidson Films, Inc., Davis, CA)

Felitti, V. (2004). The relationship of adverse childhood experiences to adult health: Turning gold into lead. Retrieved January 28, 2004, from http://www.fpc.wa .gov/relationship/adverse/childhood/experience/adult/health.pdf

Goleman, D. (1995). *Emotional intelligence*. New York: Bantam.

Kaplan, F. (2000). *Art, science and art therapy*. London: Jessica Kingsley.

Klorer, G. (2005). Expressive therapy with severely maltreated children: Neuroscience contributions. *Art Therapy: Journal of the American Art Therapy Association, 2*(4), 213–220.

Lambert, D., Bramwell, M., & Lawther, G. (1982). *The brain: A user's manual*. New York: Perigee.

LeDoux, J. (1996). *The emotional brain: The mysterious underpinnings of emotional life*. New York: Simon & Schuster.

Lusebrink, V. (1990). *Imagery and visual expression in therapy*. New York: Plenum Press.

Neufeldt, V., & Guralnik, D. B. (Eds.). (1966). *Webster's new world dictionary, college edition*. Cleveland: World.

Parnell, L. (2006 in press). *A therapist's guide to EMDR: Tools and techniques for successful treatment.* New York: W. W. Norton.

Rubenstein, S. (2006, June 11). Abandoned as a baby, now she's a graduate. *San Francisco Chronicle,* p. B3.

Schore, A. (1997). Early organization of the nonlinear right brain and development of a predisposition to psychiatric disorders. *Development and Psychopathology, 9,* 595–631.

Schore, A. (2003). Early relational trauma, disorganized attachment, and the development of a predisposition to violence. In M. Solomon and D. Siegel (Eds.), *Healing trauma* (pp. 107–167). New York: W. W. Norton.

Siegel, D. (1999). *The developing mind: Toward a neurobiology of interpersonal experience.* New York: Guilford Press.

Siegel, D. (2003). An interpersonal neurobiology of psychotherapy: The developing mind and the resolution of trauma. In M. Solomon and D. Siegel (Eds.), *Healing trauma* (pp. 1–56). New York: W. W. Norton.

Siegel, D., & Hartzell, M. (2003). *Parenting from the inside out: How a deeper self understanding can help you raise children who thrive.* Los Angeles: Tarcher Penguin.

Solomon, M., & Siegel, D. (Eds.). (2003). *Healing trauma.* New York: W. W. Norton.

van der Kolk, B., McFarlane, A., & Weisath, L. (Eds.). (1996). *Traumatic stress: The effects of overwhelming experience on mind, body, and society.* New York: Guilford Press.

Chapter 3

PATTERNS OF ATTACHMENT

Doris Banowsky Arrington and Araea Rachel Cherry

Dedicated to the children and adults who have shared their lives and
trauma in both graphic and verbal narratives.

Wired for Connection

In 2003, the Commission on Children at Risk, a panel of 33 leading
children's doctors, neuroscientists, research scholars, and youth service professionals, drew upon a large body of recent research indicating
that children and adolescents are biologically primed or *hardwired*
through enduring connections to others not only for attachment but for
moral and spiritual meaning as well. Researchers identified poor parenting in Rhesus monkeys as a precedent to deviant behavior and a
predictor of social failure. The authors introduced a new public policy
and social science term–*authoritative communities*–to describe the essential traits across social institutions that produce better outcomes for children (Commission on Children at Risk, 2003).

There is no I without a we. From a human child's beginning, he or
she is always in relationship (Arrington, 2001). Children learn that they
are valued through being cared for and enjoyed by their parental figures, and they learn how to behave when they are infants, young children, and adolescents by watching their parental figures model actions
that reflect their values. Early life experiences, notes Perry (1997), mold
and shape the core neurological organization of human beings. They
"alter connections, directly changing and forming brain structure"
(Siegel & Hartzell, 2003, p. 22). Fosha tells us that the growth of a
baby's brain requires "brain to brain interaction" (2003, p. 203).

Throughout history, human development has depended on positive interactive domains (physical, cognitive, affective, social, and spiritual) within humanity's only container, the body/mind, to move a human through what Erikson (1950) describes as the eight ages of man.[1] This chapter will briefly address the necessity of human attachment between children, age 0–5, and their primary caretakers, for trust and healthy long-term human development. It will also review the art and behavior of both securely and insecurely attached children, adolescents, and adults.

Attachment

The key figure in the area of attachment, John Bowlby, (1982), was the first to theorize that children are pre-wired for attachment. He contends that a deep and enduring relationship relating to both safety and security develops between the primary caregiver, most often, mother and child. Briere (2002) calls this a "mutual regulatory system" (p. 1). Siegel (1999) believes that "attachment relationships are the major environmental factors that shape the development of the brain during its period of maximal growth" (p. 85). Research agrees, noting that this mutual regulatory system unfolds when activated by certain cues and conditions from either the mother or the infant. A mother who provides a fragile infant with consistent feelings of safety through sensory experiences of gentle touch, warm liquid, a motherese voice, and presence, build core states of well-being while reducing anxiety, fears, sadness, and stress. Such a mother assists the infant's soft, malleable brain in forming cortical systems that regulate emotions, self-soothe, and establish trust and safety (Briere, 2002; Perry, 1994). Over time, the attachment process influences both participants. Patterns learned in the attachment phase set the base for a lifetime world view.

The brain of an infant who lacks this early caring relationship will have great difficulty in later life establishing the necessary patterns that form lasting, loving, and caring relationships with others and in developing a conscience, being authentically affectionate, and allowing anyone else to be in control (Levy & Orans, 1998). Early care is essential to this tiny human infant, an inherently social creature with behaviors that encourage acceptance and survival. He clucks, clings, sucks, smiles,

---

1. This chapter will refer to it as the eight ages of humankind.

cries, and gazes at his mother out of a basic need to woo her and to keep her close. The infant's memory of his feelings about the previous ways mother reacted will affect his future behavior (Siegel, 1999). Did mother come close so that he could smell her personal fragrance? Did she touch him or give him something warm and tasty to drink? When the child's social repertoire of success activates mother's closeness, it will also promote within the baby feelings of self-worth and security.

Bonding patterns of intimacy such as feeding, diapering, bedtime, and play between child and mother biologically encode the infant throughout the entire body. When the process is repeated and mother's behavior meets the infant's needs consistently, the prefrontal cortices (cognition) and limbic system's structures (feelings) mix with neuro-transmitters to form implicit sensory memory (i.e., it felt good, she is good, I am good). "Neural image representations" (i.e., mother, food, touch, love) are biological modifications, created by learning in a neuron circuit. They become images in our mind and precursors to eventual thoughts (i.e., mother, food, life, or self are good) (Damasio, 1994; Siegel, 1999, p. 90).

During stressful times, when children are fearful, fatigued, or ill, biochemical levels of serotonin decrease, resulting in irritability, aggression, neediness, and possibly a suppressed immune system. Because children are social beings with profound biopsychological needs for contact, comfort, nurturance, and love, sustained neglect can result in painful feelings of what appear to be deprivation and abandonment. Early acts of omission and commission actually affect the brain, serving as an etiologic reservoir for the development of later psychological disorders (Briere, 2002, p. 2). This includes children of all ages who live in conflictual households or neighborhoods in which there are high levels of hostility. They often respond in kind. If they are very young, they may freeze in fear (Arrington & Cherry, 2004). If they are older they may react aggressively, and if they are old enough to be able to, they will flee, taking with them their abusive experiences and internalized aggressive role models (Bell & Jenkins, 1993). Noting the strong relationship between child abuse and neglect and early-onset violence, prostitution, and substance abuse, psychologists see few possibilities that these victimized insecurely attached children will not also abuse their children and spouses (Glicken, 2004).

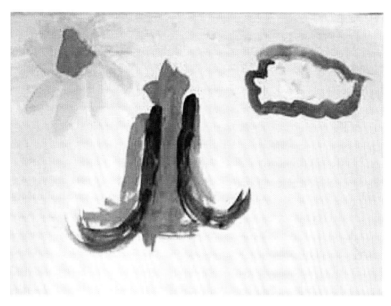

Figure 3.1. *The Volcano,* by Howard, an angry 8-year-old.

Howard was filled with anger and rage. During a potent puppet play session with his art therapist, Howard was filled with violence and aggression toward the therapist's puppet. He spoke to the intergenerational effects of family violence. Yelling at the puppet, he said, "Oh yes, I do have to hurt you! My grandpa hurt my daddy, my daddy hurt me, and I am going to hurt my kids!" Howard is already programmed to be an abuser.

Volcanoes are a popular metaphor for feelings of anger and rage. Howard painted this following the construction of two separate clay volcanoes. Howard could not rest until he filled each of the clay volcanoes with red paint. Just filling the volcanoes with paint did not adequately portray his anger and rage, so at the art therapist's suggestion he plunged the paint inside the volcanoes up and down with a paintbrush handle to make it flow out of the volcanoes' cinder cones. "I need lots of paint," he said. He plunged and plunged and plunged, making angry sounds all the while.

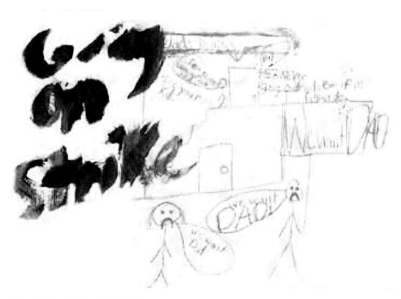

Figure 3.2. *Father's Day,* by Wesley, a 10-year-old boy reacting to an absent father on Father's Day.

Wesley, generally calm and playful, was enraged and aggressive. Father's Day was coming up and he was aware there was no way that he would see the father he hardly knew, nor his mother, who was in rehabilitation in another city after serving jail time for drug possession. First, he picked up play guns in the playroom and shot his brother, who was also in the session, and the therapist. When he was offered art materials, his usual noninterest in art disappeared and he begin drawing and telling the therapist in a loud voice what was going on in his picture. "We want Dad! We want Dad! We want Dad! Please come outside and see your kids. NO! I'm never going outside even if it is Father's Day."

Wesley picked up paints and began mixing red and black paint, using it to write "On Strike," smearing the paint on himself and the table. Encouraging him to continue painting, the therapist gave him more paper. He filled the second paper with paint and then folded it over, where it dried together. Wesley, with two absent parents, is a youngster imprinted with loss and insecurity. Without appropriate interventions, he will face a lifetime of aggressive and defensive maneuvers.

Attachment is best understood by observing a young child, who after having developed a secure base with the primary mother figure, can leave the attachment figure to explore his surroundings for longer and longer periods of time. The opposite occurs with children who have experienced chronic separation and deprivation (Ainsworth, Blehar, Waters, & Wall, 1978). As a result of a child being insecurely attached, or having experienced avoidant, resistant, or disorganized attachment, he/she cannot meet biological needs of exploration and will develop an ongoing sense of anxiety, frustration, and self-recrimination (Levy & Orlans, 1998). This separation conflict will permanently affect the infant's cognitive, physiological, social, and spiritual health domains, playing a role in later thoughts, feelings, and memories (Siegel, 1999).

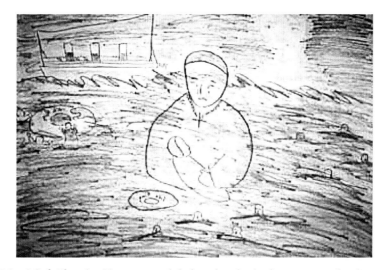

Figure 3.3. *A Safe Place,* by Nancy, an adult female who had experienced a deep trauma.

Attachment, a deep and enduring tie established between a child (infant) and caregiver (mother) in the first years of life, is a basic human need rooted in human existence. This secure base, sought out by children during periods of stress or alarm, "sets the stage for the exploratory behavior that allows an individual to be productive and autonomous" (Frances, Kaiser, & Deaver, 2003, p. 125). The internalized attachment model profoundly influences every component of the human condition—mind, body, emotions, relationships, and values. This internal process produces a myriad of behaviors that among other things identifies a child's readiness for formal learning. These behaviors include capacities for conscious attention, perseverance, curiosity, optimism, initiative, service, resilience, confidence, self-control, communication, humor, courage, and empathy and cooperation. In addition, conscious attention (explicit memory) is required for encoding of perception through sight, sound, touch, taste, hearing, and conception (ideas, notions, and theory) (Seigel & Hartzell, 2003).

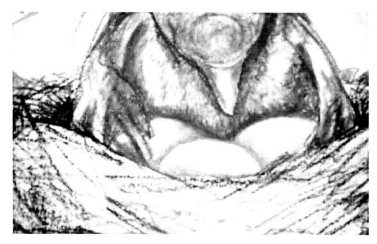

Figure 3.4. Bird Nest, drawing by Yoko, a mother who had securely attached to her children.

From a child's earliest child-parent relationship, the internal working models or core-relational schemas formed are based on "beliefs that function more as a general model of self and others than as actual thoughts" (Briere, 2002, p. 2). These core schemas, both cognitive and emotional, narrative and graphic, affect the individual's capacity to live fully with trust and meaningful attachments with others. The more care or lack of care an experience-dependent infant and toddler receives, the more he or she will remember how to respond in kind. A child insecurely attached because of neglect and a lack of love will have limited memories of what love feels like and how he or she should react to love and kindness throughout his or her entire life.

Implicit Memory

As infants experience sensations, emotions, feelings, and perceptions, specific patterns of interactions and behavior encode implicit memories

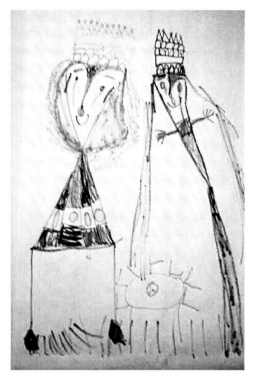

Figure 3.5. *Me and My Sister,* by Haley, a 5-year-old child from a secure home.

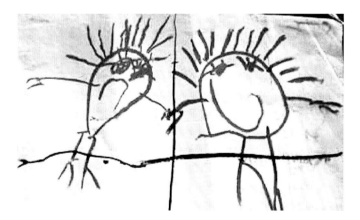

Figure 3.6. *My Sister's Sad,* by Kelly, a 5-year-old child from a violent home.

in the brain, i.e., procedural memories that are nonverbal, nonautobiographical, and nontime oriented, such as behaviors, habits, skills, gestures, postures, and imaged memories associated with "safety or danger,
such as sounds, darkness, smells, visual images and body states"
(Kozlowska & Hanney, 2001, p. 51). These primal psychobiological
experiences (1) *encode* in the brain and the body. The brain (2) *stores*
cues about the event, i.e., what was seen, how it felt, smelled, tasted, or
sounded. When similar sensate cues indicate to the brain that the body
is in a similar environment, the brain (3) *retrieves* the event in implicit
memory patterns. These early, self-perpetuating patterns form the base
for repeated behaviors out of which explicit memory builds. Therefore,
having a parent who has highly developed parental meta-emotional
philosophy, one who is high in knowing and responding to his or her
own emotions and discussing emotional responses with the children
helps children learn to regulate impulsive behavior and self-soothe
when upset (Katz-Fainsilber, 2006).

In the first 2–3 years of development, implicit patterns are the property of the relationship between caregiver and child. It is significant to note
that if the primary caregiver changes, the pattern will have an opportunity to make some change. After three to five years of age, implicit patterns are the property of the child and change is unlikely even if the
parent's parenting skills improve later (Bowlby, 1982). The critical time
period for establishing this secure base model is by the age of five.

Developmental researchers, building on the work of Bowlby (1982),
Ainsworth et al. (1978), and Main and Goldwyn (1984–1998), report that
the attachment process, as outlined above, serves as a blueprint for *all*
future relationships (Briere, 2002; Perry, 1999). Emphasizing "the growing awareness in cognitive-behavioral circles," Briere (2002) observes
"implicit memories and processes are–at minimum–as important as
explicit ones, and that emotion is as important as cognition in understanding and treating anxiety-based disorders" (p. 1). Of critical interest
to both medical and mental health clinicians is that "the factual knowledge required for reasoning and decision making, including words and
abstract symbols, comes to the mind in the form of images" (p. 96). For
example, if the Golden Gate Bridge is mentioned and you cross it daily,
you will have a myriad of thoughts, perhaps pleasant or unpleasant,
interacting with a collage of images that relate to it, from its size, people
walking on it (visual), cars driving on it (auditory), the fog or sun on it
(affect) and perhaps even articles you have read about it (cognitive).

The following pictures are from Cherry's work with children who lived with their moms in the shelter for women who had experienced domestic violence where Cherry worked for over ten years. These children know sadness and depression. Their mothers know fear.

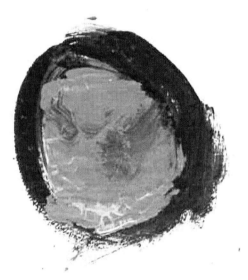

Figure 3.7. *This Is My Heart All Covered Up. To Uncover It Will Take a Lot of Education* by Olivia, age 6.

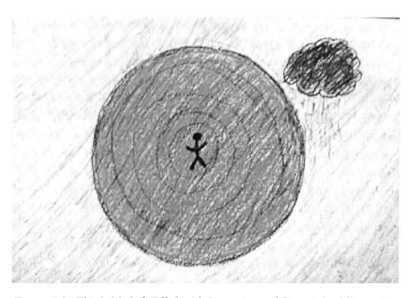

Figure 3.8. *This Is My Life Filled with Depression and Despair,* by Jill, age 14.

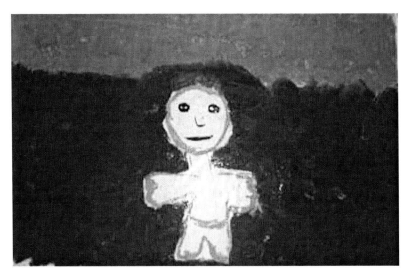

Figure 3.9. *Something I Am Sad About,* by Bobby, age 7.

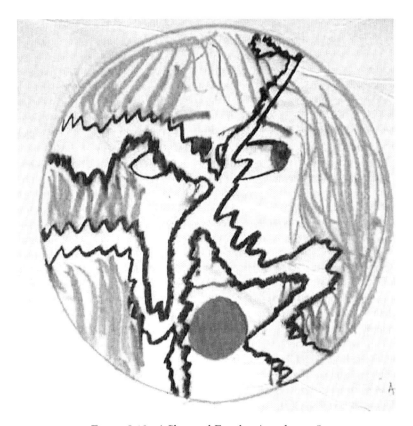

Figure 3.10. *A Shattered Face,* by Angel, age 9.

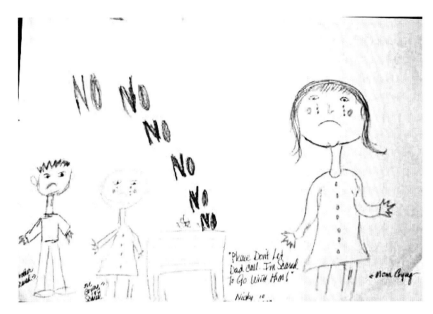

Figure 3.11. *No! No! No! I Don't Want Daddy to Call,* by Carrie, an 11-year-old in the domestic violence shelter with her mother.

Explicit Memory

"Explicit memory," different from implicit memory, "is concerned with distinct facts and a person's conscious awareness of knowing them" (Sapolsky, 1998, p. 175). For a toddler, explicit memory begins with autobiographical information and timing. This can be seen in a first memory, i.e., a three-year-old's memory of her mother bringing a baby sibling home from the hospital (obviously an emotional trigger). When implicit and explicit memories mix, they can dramatically affect thoughts and behavior. Memory, fact, and feeling can create childhood fantasies that can persist into adulthood or beyond.

Example: Ann. Ann, born at home, was sent at age ten to live for six months with relatives when her mother had a hysterectomy. In her thirties, while discussing her birth story with her therapist, she mixed implicit and explicit memories. Ann always felt guilty, believing that she deserved to be sent away from the family because by being born at home instead of in a hospital she had caused her mother's illness. In her own mind, she had fantasized the home as being dark and not as sterile as the hospital, preventing treatment from being adequately hygienic. In fact, the doctor had recommended home birth because he felt the home would be more sterile.

Secure Patterns of Attachment

At approximately age seven months, regions of the brain establish patterns of attachment. With most children, these patterns become securely established around 36 months. Secure patterns of attachment to their mothers allow children to move out into the world to explore and develop relationships with others (Ainsworth et al., 1978), unlike the poorly attached child with few to no social skills. Stable patterns of social control such as internalized models of self-soothing and emotional self-control provide the child with behavioral skills that allow him to be accepted and to survive successfully within his developing social environment.

Stages of Attachment

Bowlby (1982) identified four stages a child goes through if separated from his/her primary caregiver. Anyone that has been around a child for any period of time will recognize them.

- **Protest**—an expression of pain and yearning for the primary object, mother. The child displays his alarm.
- **Despair**—When mother still does not return, the child, wanting to get rid of the pain and despair, cries and cries without relief.
- **Detachment**—The child takes the position of "I will no longer care" because the pain of separation hurts too much.
- **Reorganization**—When the child has relinquished all hope that the lost mother will be recovered, the child looks for a way to survive and once again feel secure. The emotional affect flattens and the child moves into the final stage of reorganization.

An unstable, chaotic environment prevents a child from attending to the developmental task of childhood of developing a sense of self. Distortion of self-image is one of the most devastating effects of family abuse. Young children seen by art therapists commonly exhibit low self-esteem with feelings of inadequacy and inferiority. The art or play therapist has a pivotal relationship with a child who has low self-esteem. She helps the child complete certain developmental tasks, acquire a sense of independence, and learn about his or her strengths and capabilities through the use of art materials. She also helps children learn to self-soothe and regulate impulsive behavior when they get upset.

When Matty completed her painting, she stepped back, pointed proudly at her picture, and with flashing eyes and a huge grin, exclaimed: "That's me!"

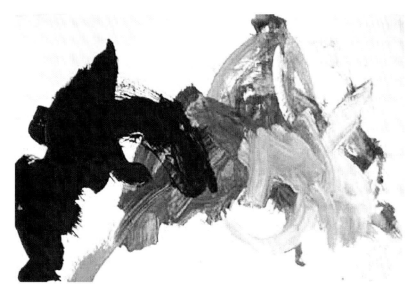

Figure 3.12. *That's me!* by Matty, age 3. Patterns of Infant Strange Situation Behavior.

Ainsworth collaborated with Bowlby on his work on attachment at Tavistock Clinic in England in the 1950s. Later, intending to illuminate the infant's attachment system, Ainsworth studied mother-child interactions through observation of a separation-reunion experience. Ainsworth's study has been replicated many times. It separates and reunites a one-year-old from his/her attachment figure within a strange environment. Called the Ainsworth or Infant Strange Situation (ISS) test, it is coded with the self-soothing and return-to-play behavior of the infant as the child seeks proximity to the attachment figure. The most instructive part of the study was the reunion. Here, Ainsworth and her students were able to codify distinct reunion patterns. This instrument has been recognized as the most consistent predictor of how "infants become or will become attached to their parents" (Siegel, 1999, p. 81).

Ainsworth's Patterns of Infant Strange Situation Behavior are:

• **Secure Attachment**–Misses parent during separation but calms down and returns to play when parent returns;

- **Avoidant Attachment**–Avoids or ignores parent on return; focus on toys, not parent;
- **Resistant or Ambivalent Attachment**–Preoccupied with parent, not toys or environment;
- **Disorganized or Disoriented Attachment**–May freeze, cling, cry, or lean away. (Ainsworth et al., 1978)

In the 1980s, Ainsworth's students, Main and Goldwyn, developed an analysis of the Adult Attachment Interview (AAI) that assessed the mental process of the parent. They "found that secure versus insecure childhood attachment status, as observed in Ainsworth's Infant's Strange Situation, can often predict later adult attachment findings" (Seigel, 1999, p. 78). Siegel (1999) reports that the 45- to 90-minute interview with a stranger contained questions about the parent's own childhood similar to: "What was it like to grow up in your family?" "What experiences did you have that were upsetting, threatening, or fearful?" "How have your early experiences shaped your parenting style today?" "Give five adjectives for each of your parents." The Main/Goldwyn analysis leads to ratings of what is called the "current state of mind" with respect to attachment (Seigel, 1999, p. 79). The AAI analysis materials include an important request that the participants (1) be truthful, (2) provide evidence of what they say, (3) be relevant, and (4) be clear and orderly (Grice, as cited by Siegel 1999, p. 80).

Ainsworth (1978) found, through her work with children and their mothers, that children develop mental models of themselves, others, and life in general, i.e., "I am good or bad, nice or mean, loved or unloved, beautiful or ugly, responsible or irresponsible, "The world is safe or dangerous; people are trustworthy or not trustworthy," etc., through both family and environment (peaceful vs. violent communities). These influences build internal attachment patterns that become core beliefs, anticipatory images, or world views that influence the individual throughout life. Young children do not blame their problems on their parents or the world outside; instead, they imagine that they themselves are bad and have done something wrong, as did Ann, who believed she had caused her mother's illness (Oaklander, 1978).

Figures 3.13-3.15 are drawings by three adults in a domestic violence shelter in response to the question, "How do you feel?"

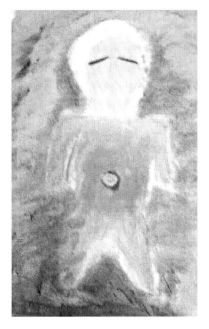

Figure 3.13. *Frozen in Fear.*

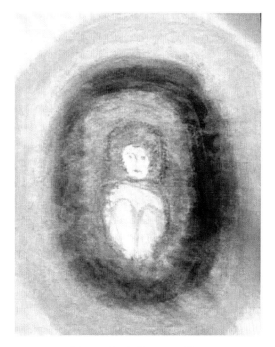

Figure 3.14. *Frozen in Fear.*

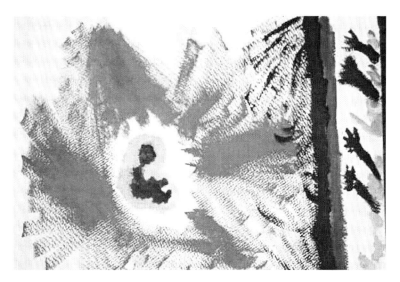

Figure 3.15. *Frozen in Fear.*

Disrupted Attachment

Children whose brains cells have sensed, perceived, and acted on information gathered in an environment of abuse, neglect, and other adverse childhood experiences are organized to survive in toxic environments. Felitti, one of the core researchers of the Adverse Childhood Experiences study, notes, "A child does not just get over some things, not even 50 years later. Childhood experiences affect adult health decades later" (2004, p. 1).

Children raised by unresponsive or otherwise emotionally neglectful and absent parents "appear to be at risk for psychological disturbances in the short, intermediate, and in the long term as well," says Hudd (2002, p. 179).

Example: Molly. Molly, a senior, had been left on the church steps when she was an infant. Although when she was a child, a family cared for her with their other children, she was never legally adopted or treated as one of their own. She married a caring, attentive man and they had two happy children, but most of her adult physical and emotional life was spent with psychosomatic illnesses and obsessive-compulsive behavior; she was unable to handle even small changes well. Her nuclear family learned to nurture her illnesses and to live with her anxieties. As she grew older and her husband died, she became more dependent and anxious, unable to find or remember any self-soothing remedies.

Disrupted and anxious attachment leads not only to emotional distress and social problems but also results in biochemical consequences in the developing brain. Infants raised with limited touch and security have abnormally high levels of stress hormones (Perry, 1994). The neurobiological consequences for these children are seen in a lack of ability to self-regulate (lack of impulse control) and in psychosocial problems such as physical and sexual aggression against themselves and others.

Children with disrupted attachment disorder, identified as reactive attachment disorder (RAD), have difficulties forming lasting and loving relationships, developing a conscience, trusting, being authentically affectionate, or allowing anyone else to be in control. RAD is caused by any kind of abuse (physical, emotional, or sexual), neglect, sudden separation from a primary caregiver (due to illness, death, or travel), undiagnosed or painful illness, inconsistent or inadequate care, chronically depressed caregivers, a variety of moves or home placements as in foster care or multiple marriages by a parent, as well as care providers with limited caregiving skills.

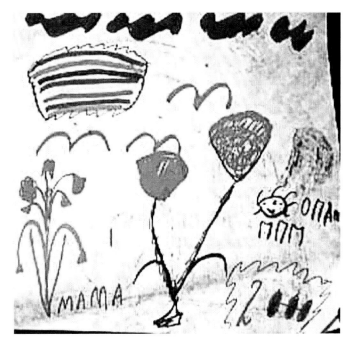

Figure 3.16. *A free drawing* by Moisha, a disrupted attached 5-year-old.

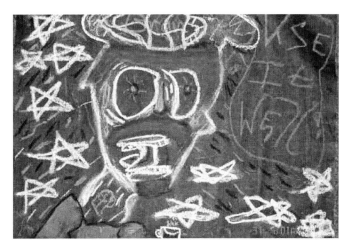

Figure 3.17. *The Brain, Use it Well,* by James, a traumatized 10-year-old.

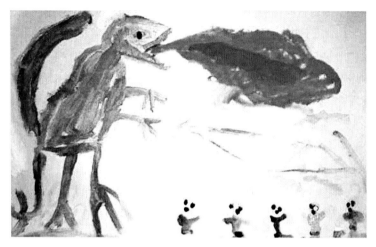

Figure 3.18. *A Family Portrait* by Terry, a disrupted attached teenager.

An art therapy group with children from violent or unsafe homes includes ground rules and clear limits designed to avoid activating traumatizing memories. These rules include the following:

LISTEN and ENCOURAGE them to talk about their feelings.
GIVE OPTIONS for taking care of themselves.
BE HONEST.
RECOGNIZE positive actions or behaviors.
EXPLORE their interests.
MODEL HAVING FUN by singing, dancing, playing, making art, acting, and writing poetry.
INCORPORATE storytelling, guided imagery, and books for kids.
DRAW and talk about the pictures.
PLAY GAMES, solve problems.
TEACH kids how to be a friend.
SMILE a lot and encourage lots of God Hugs (Butterfly hugs).

Conclusion

"Attachment is an inborn system in the brain that evolves in ways that influence and organize motivational, emotional and memory process with respect to significant caregiving figures" (Bowlby, as cited by Siegel, 1999, p. 67). Mother and Daddy are the first objects of the child's attention. Their responses are the true Toys "R" Us™ (fun and games) experience for their children (Glasser & Easley, 1998). From their parents' acceptance or rejection, children learn behavior. From their parents' early communication patterns of touch and tone, children learn trust. Repeated behaviors in significant relationships early in life shape the structural developments of the infant and child's brain. As we have seen earlier, those parenting behaviors form the child's world view that last a lifetime.

"Affective change processes, however, are naturally occurring phenomena. They reflect how we are wired" (Fosha, 2003, p. 232). It is encouraging to note that whereas adults may have grown up with parents who were "preoccupied" or "dismissing" or "disorganized," resulting in their not being securely based, Fosha points out that "transformational effects operate not only in therapy but in development" (2003, p. 232) in love or student-teacher relationships, in friendships, or in religious experiences, resulting in adults finding a secure base, a safe haven to self-soothe when upset and a way to understand their life stories. These state-of-mind attunements are encouraged and supported through both verbal and nonverbal communication methods such as caring eye contact, warm voice tone, and reaching out bodily movements.

Today, more and more programs include many ways of communicating and helping both parents and their children communicate about their feelings. Meta-emotion intervention programs aimed at helping parents talk to their children about emotions as well as discussing parental beliefs and attitudes about emotions assist parents and children in developmental attachment tasks (Katz & Gottman, 1991).

References

Ainsworth, M. D., Blehar, M. C., Waters, E., & Wall, S. (1978). *Patterns of attachment: A psychological study of the strange situation.* Hillsdale, NJ: Erlbaum.

Arrington, D. B. (2001). *Home is where the art is: An art therapy approach to family therapy.* Springfield, IL: Charles C Thomas.

Arrington, D. B., & Cherry, R. (2004). Long-term intergenerational affects of violent families: Frozen in fear. In *35th Proceedings of the American Art Therapy Association* (p. 134). San Diego, CA: American Art Therapy Association.

Bell, C. C., & Jenkins, E. J. (1993). Community violence and children on Chicago's south side. *Psychiatry, 56,* 46–54.

Bowlby, J. (1982). *Attachment and loss. Vol. 1: Attachment* (2nd ed.). New York: Basic Books.

Briere, J. (2002). Treating adult survivors of severe childhood abuse and neglect: Further developments of an integrative model. In J. E. Meyers, L. Berlinger, J. Briere, C.T. Hendrix, T. Reid, & C. Jenny (Eds.), *The APSAC Handbook on child maltreatment* (2nd ed.). Newbury Park, CA: Sage Publications.

Commission on Children at Risk. (2003). *Hardwired to connect: The new scientific case for authoritative communities.* Executive summary. Retrieved February 26, 2006, from http://www.americanvalues.org/html/hardwired.html

Erikson, E. (1963). *Childhood and society* (2nd ed.). New York: W. W. Norton.

Damasio, A. (1994). *Descartes' error: Emotion, reason and the human brain.* New York: Avon.

Felitti, V. (2004). *The relationship of adverse childhood experiences to adult health: Turning gold into lead.* Retrieved January 28, 2004, from http://www.fpc.wa.gov/relationship/adverse/childhood/experience/adult/health.pdf

Fosha, D. (2003). Dyadic regulation and experiential work with emotion and relatedness in trauma and disorganized attachment. In M. Solomon & D. Siegel (Eds.), *Healing trauma: Attachment, mind, body, and brain* (pp. 1–56.) New York: W. W. Norton.

Frances, D., Kaiser D., & Deaver, D. (2003). Representations of attachment security in the bird's nest drawings of clients with substance abuse disorders. *Art Therapy: Journal of the American Art Therapy Association 20*(3), 123-124.

Glasser, H., & Easley, J. (1998). *Transforming the difficult child: The nurtured heart approach.* Tucson, AZ: Author. Available from adhddoc@the river.com.

Glicken, M. (2004). *Violent young children.* Boston: Pearson Education.

Hudd, S. (2002). Finding the way back home: Children's story of family attachment. In A. Cattanach (Ed.), *The story so far* (pp. 149–186). London: Jessica Kingsley.

Katz, L. & Gottman, J. (1991). Marital discord and child outcomes: A social psychophysiological approach. In K. Dodge & J. Garber (Eds.), *The development of emotion regulation and deregulation.* New York: Cambridge University.

Katz-Fainsilber, L. (2006). Domestic violence, emotion coaching, and child adjustment. *Journal of Family Psychology, 20*(1), 56–67.

Kozlowska, K., & Hanney, L. (2001). An art therapy group for children traumatized by parental violence and separation. *Clinical Child Psychology and Psychiatry, 6*(1), 49–78.

Levy, T., & Orlans, M. (1998). *Attachment, trauma and healing: Understanding and treating attachment disorder in children and families.* Washington, DC: Child Welfare League of America Press.

Main, M., & Goldwyn, R. (1984–1998). *Adult attachment scoring and classification system.* Unpublished manuscript, Department of Psychology, University of California at Berkeley.

Oaklander, V. (1978). *Windows to our children.* Moab, UT: Real People.

Perry, B. (1994). Neurobiological sequelae of childhood trauma: Posttraumatic stress in children. Retrieved September 6, 2006, from http://www.childtrauma.org/cta-materials/ptsd_child.asp

Perry, B. (1997). Incubated in terror: Neurodevelopmental factors in the "cycle of violence." In J. Osofsky (Ed.), *Children in a violent society* (pp. 124–149). New York: Guilford Press.

Siegel, D. (1999). *The developing mind: Toward a neurobiology of interpersonal experience.* New York: Guilford Press.

Siegel, D., & Hartzell, M. (2003). *Parenting from the inside out: How a deeper self understanding can help you raise children who thrive.* Los Angeles: Tarcher Penguin.

Sapolsky, M. (1998). *Why zebras don't get ulcers: An updated guide to stress, stress-related disease and coping.* New York: W. H. Freeman.

Chapter 4

CHILDHOOD CANCER AND SURVIVORSHIP

JoAnna Wallace

*Dedicated to my mother, who is a source of strength and
inspiration in my work and life.*

In the United States, each year approximately 12,500 children are
diagnosed with cancer, a remarkable 50 children a day (Leukemia
and Lymphoma Society, 2006). Fortunately, the survival rates have
increased dramatically over the past 40 years. The majority of the children diagnosed with cancer today will be long-term survivors. Currently, approximately 70 percent–75 percent of children diagnosed with
cancer will survive (Keene, Hobbie, & Ruccione, 2000). Twenty years
ago, the focus of the medical teams was to diminish pain and to cope
with death. Today, however, the new emphasis is on survivorship and
the impending ramifications of treatment.

As the doctors continue to research and employ new treatments that
successfully decrease the mortality and morbidity of serious childhood
illnesses, the psychosocial needs of the patients have increased. The
success of survival can be bittersweet. Although the advancement in
treating childhood cancer is helping children live longer, there can be
short- and long-term effects. Childhood cancer survivors may face years
of illness, treatment, stress, and post-treatment effects. The ramifications of the operations, procedures, treatments, and medications can
leave the children battling with emotional, physical, and cognitive
effects (Last, Grootenhuis, & Eiser, 2005). As survivorship continues to
increase, therapists are needed to assist the clients in coping with the
difficulties that result from disease and treatment. Today's treatment

teams strive to meet the needs of the child and administer comprehensive treatment that incorporates mental health services.

This chapter explores the emotional aspects and developmental stages of children with cancer as they travel along the difficult journey of diagnosis, treatment, and survivorship. The chapter also demonstrates the use of art therapy to address the psychosocial needs of children with cancer, illustrates a descriptive case study, and demonstrates the benefits of a group art therapy program.

Diagnosis

The diagnosis of cancer changes a child's life forever. For most children, a precancerous life was predictable: they woke up, ate breakfast, went to school, had play dates, spent time with family, and then bedtime. With the diagnosis of cancer, a child's world is essentially placed in the spin cycle of a washing machine. The child lacks command and is randomly tossed and turned in many directions. Cancer takes away the control a child has over his or her daily life. The child lacks power as he or she is poked and prodded, and taken from the normalcy of home and school. Rather than struggling to learn their ABCs or the next math equation, children diagnosed with cancer are suddenly forced to lead an alien life coping with painful procedures, numerous medications, and hospital stays and visits.

The diagnosis of cancer can be overwhelming for a family. Many parents may want to try to protect the child from the truth of the diagnosis and illness. Most experts agree, however, that it is important for parents to communicate with their children and keep them informed, using developmentally appropriate language. It is important not to hide information and for a child to understand the illness and the treatment procedures that will be used. Research is indicating that children experience less duress from their illness and treatments when they are kept informed and given information in age-appropriate terms (Keene, Hobbie, & Ruccione, 2000; Melman & Sanders, 1986; Patenaude & Kupst, 2005; Sourkes, 1995). Learning about cancer and what to expect can help prepare a child for the challenges ahead.

Medical Treatment

Medical treatments for childhood cancer include surgery, radiation therapy, chemotherapy, and stem cell transplantation. Cancer treatment can last from several months to several years. The medical treatments for cancer can cause short and long-term physical and psychological effects. The short-term physical effects can include hair loss, nausea and vomiting, low blood count (decreased ability to fight infection), weight gain, constipation, fatigue, dental problems, mouth sores, changes in taste and smell, and skin and nail problems. Physical long-term effects can include changes in development and growth, physical limitations, effects on puberty and fertility, problems with teeth and sinuses, issues with cognitive functioning, and the development of second cancers (Hodder & Keene, 2002).

Any physical change that occurs is a constant reminder for children with cancer that they are different from other children. The psychological effects are also short- and long-term and can include fear about how the child will look and feel and how others, including friends, will react. The constant change in physical appearance and "feeling different" can cause a drop in a child's self-esteem. In one study (Ross & Ross, 1984), children with cancer reported that being made fun of about their weight gain or hair loss was worse than the physical pain they experienced from treatment.

Although procedures and treatments are usually nonnegotiable, it can often be helpful to give the child as much control as possible. It is helpful to assist children in gaining control in their external environment since they have relinquished control of their bodies. For example, a child can put on numbing cream for needles, choose a band-aid, decide the order in which to take pills, or choose a successful pill-swallowing agent (Hodder & Keene, 2002).

Furthermore, it is also important for someone on the treatment team to normalize the physical limitations and changes that occur in the child's appearance (e.g., hair loss) throughout treatment. It is often helpful for a child to meet other children experiencing similar circumstances or to read personal stories to enable the child to find comfort in the fact that he or she is not alone.

After the Cancer Experience–Late Effects

For cancer survivors, the end of treatment can bring an entirely new set of difficulties. Late effects are side effects of cancer treatment that appear in the child months or years after the treatment. Late effects can include physical, psychological, and cognitive difficulties. Ironically, the treatments that are saving so many lives are also being labeled as the cause of late effects. The toxic treatments administered during the child's time of prime development and growth has been shown to be causing long-term effects for childhood cancer survivors. The treatment that is used to kill cancer cells also attacks normal cells in the body. The severities of the side effects are related to (1) location and type of cancer, (2) age at treatment, and (3) length, type, and intensity of treatment.

Physical late effects can include changes in appearance, stunted growth and development, and physical disabilities. In addition, some children can develop problems with their heart, lungs, kidneys, fertility, hearing, and teeth (National Association of Social Workers & Children's Cause Cancer Advocacy, 2006).

The emotional impact of surviving cancer can be very complex. Psychological problems can include feelings of grief or loss of the normalcy of childhood. The children can experience general psychological distress including social anxiety, poor peer acceptance, and self-perception issues (Bessell, 2001). There may also be symptoms of posttraumatic stress due to painful memories, reminders of stressful events, or the fear of relapse.

Common cognitive late effects include slowed thinking or processing speed, attention problems, memory difficulties, fine motor problems, difficulty planning and organizing tasks and materials, poor handwriting, poor reading comprehension, and poor math skills. When cognitive deficits appear, damage has occurred to the brain and slowed down its processing ability, making it difficult for new connections of new brain development to occur (Sumpter, 2005). Baseline and post-treatment neuropsychological evaluation is recommended for children at higher risk for cognitive problems.

Development

The child with cancer experiences a detour or obstacle to the path of "normal development" due to the medical treatment used to rid the body of cancer. Illness at any time during childhood can cause a regression or conflict in development. For example, a sick child who achieved independence and previously slept in her own bed may demand to sleep with her parents at night. Children who are hospitalized for the majority of their young lives may exhibit deficits in their ability to play with peers due to a lack of experience and exposure.

According to Erikson (1963), when a child is approximately three to six years old, he or she is considered to be in the stage of learning initiative versus guilt. During this stage, children learn (1) to imagine, and to increase their skills through play and fantasy, (2) to cooperate with others, and (3) to be leaders as well as followers. It is important for a child in this developmental stage to develop trust with adults. A child who is in the hospital is challenged to attain a basic sense of trust. The young child is often separated from parents and may be deprived of sufficient bonding time. The child may also view adults as people who inflict pain and duress. The child may be too young to make the connection between a painful procedure and future health (Eiser, 2004). According to Erikson (1963), the child who is mistrusting will doubt the future and will experience defeat and feelings of inferiority.

Erikson labeled ages six to 12 as the industry versus inferiority stage. During this stage, children learn to master life skills: (1) social relationships with peers, (2) teamwork, and (3) social studies, reading, and arithmetic. The child's development during this stage involves attaining autonomy and relationships with friends. Children with cancer, however, are often restricted from normal play with peers due to hospitalizations or immunosuppression. Treatment for cancer can isolate a child, cause a child to feel different, and create difficulties in maintaining friendships (Eiser, 2004). In addition, latency-age children are old enough to pick up on their parents' anxieties and worries. The medically fragile child might repress true feelings of anger and fear. The child may take on a parentified role and attempt to shield her parents from the hurt her illness may cause them. The child may also feel guilty or responsible for causing stress in the family and try to make up for it in a myriad of ways. Cancer challenges a child's ability to attain and maintain autonomy and friendships.

Erikson (1963) labeled adolescence the stage of learning identity versus role confusion. According to Erikson, during successful adolescence, the key developmental steps include independence from family, development of a supportive peer group, and the establishment of work and career goals. Cancer challenges the achievement of adolescent developmental goals. Adolescents suffering from cancer may be forced to be dependent on their parents and can miss out on a normal social life (Eiser, 2004). Furthermore, adolescents are highly concerned about their appearance. Changes in physical appearance due to medical treatment may result in poor body image and lack of self-worth, and may affect relationships. Adolescents with cancer risk being unable to attain Erikson's developmental stages of identity and intimacy.

Cancer challenges the normal sequence of developmental stages. Reengaging a child back into activities in school and with friends, as soon as medically possible, is the best way to minimize disruptions in a child's development (Keene, Hobbie, & Ruccione, 2000).

Art Therapy and Treatment

For many years, art has been a developmentally appropriate means for working with children with cancer (Lusebrink, 1990). In the medical setting, art therapy provides tactile stimulation, nonverbal communication, an opportunity for choice, and a means to achieve control (Appleton, 2001; Councill, 1993; Malchiodi, 1999). The art therapy session provides a safe place to use media and the creative process to express emotions. The art therapist uses the art product to provide the patient-artist with insight into his inner and outer thoughts and feelings. In addition, the simplicity of creating can build confidence and promote positive self-esteem. A recent study with adult cancer patients found that art therapy was also effective in reducing pain symptoms (Nainis et al., 2006).

Art is a familiar language for all children, and for the child with cancer, often what cannot be said in words can be said through images. The art product, a concrete product, when used as an assessment tool can be presented to the medical team to assist in the communication of the child's emotional status and response to her illness and treatment (Teufel, 1995).

Individual and Group Art Therapy

The art therapy program I have developed focuses on meeting the needs of children battling cancer. My work provides support for the child and the family throughout medical treatment and survivorship. Art therapy assists a child with cancer in coping with the physical illness, treatment procedures, and psychological issues associated with cancer. The child finds an art therapy session to provide both a safe place and a means to express her feelings and experiences. For children suffering with cancer, I work in both an individual and group art therapy format. The individual art therapy services offer specialized support addressing the child's current difficulties, stressors, and needs. The art therapy group provides opportunities for children with cancer to interact and learn ways to cope, and reduces fear and anxiety.

It is important to note that there may be limitations when working with this medically fragile population. Children with cancer may have physical limitations such as fatigue and loss of mobility as well as emotional stress, and they may frequently miss appointments due to illness or medical procedures. Furthermore, some children, due to the risk of infection, will require new or sterilized materials.

The following is a case study of a young girl with a diagnosis of leukemia.

Case Study: Alexis

Alexis, diagnosed with leukemia at age four, began art therapy treatment after she experienced anxiety around medical procedures, self-consciousness about physical changes, and being teased at school about her looks. Her family, supportive and nurturing, recognized Alexis's need for psychosocial support. Alexis, a very creative child whose drawing ability was above her developmental level, enjoyed drawing and creating artwork. Art therapy was a good match.

Stuyck (2003) argues that children are more likely to express themselves spontaneously through pictures than through a strictly verbal discussion with a therapist. Rollins (2005) postulates that art therapists use art to enhance the child's ability to communicate through visual expression and verbal response to their images. Alexis used art to depict her medical experiences and difficulties. The art acted as a springboard for dialogue with her parents, the medical team, and me.

For example, Alexis used drawing as an outlet to depict her "needle" pokes to gain control, to release frustration, and to plan coping strategies for the pain (Figures 4.1 and 4.2). Alexis would draw her images and then explain the picture. I would then make further inquiries, provide a holding environment, and assisting in problem solving.

Figure 4.1 is an image Alexis drew at the age of four of receiving a needle "poke" from a nurse. The picture is drawn with a smiling nurse standing over the bed with large hands, while Alexis is in the bed with a frown and a spot on her hand to represent the "ouch." Alexis verbally expressed feelings of pain and sadness about receiving pokes. In addition, Alexis assumed that the nurse enjoyed giving her the needle

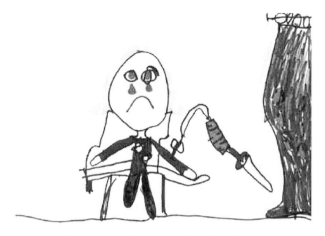

Figure 4.1. *Receiving a Poke,* by Alexis.

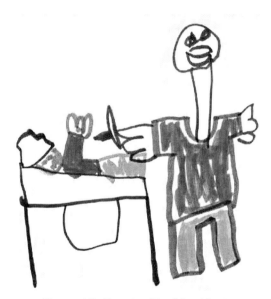

Figure 4.2. *Drawing Blood,* by Alexis.

and that receiving the needle poke was about something Alexis had done wrong. I worked with Alexis to reassure her she had done nothing wrong to receive the needles and that the nurses did not want to hurt children but to help children get better.

Figure 4.2 was created one year later and is an image of a blood draw. Alexis drew herself alone, crying, with arms outstretched. In addition, the red polka dots drawn on the curtain ironically resemble blood drops. Alexis expressed feeling that she wanted to cry during blood draws but did not want to make her mom sad. Therapeutically, I was able to reassure Alexis that feeling and expressing emotions was normal, and healthy, and that her mom loved her no matter what.

Alexis's drawings often depicted scenes at school where due to her hair loss she was being teased about looking like a boy.

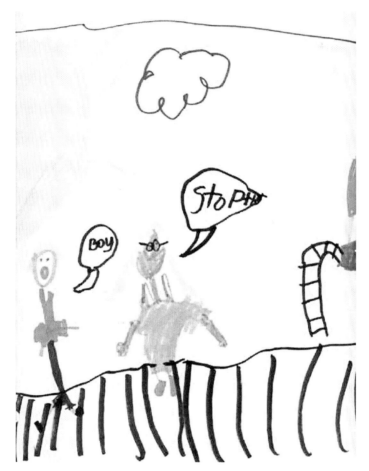

Figure 4.3. *Being Teased,* by Alexis.

Although Alexis was bald, she ironically always drew herself with long, blond hair. In addition, her hair was often depicted with embellishments and elaborate details. Through the art process, the teasing was identified as coming during recess from one particular classmate. The artwork acted as a tangible communication tool that was shared with her mother and teacher in order to address the problem and advocate for Alexis at school.

Through art, Alexis was able to gain control and to create her own solutions to parts of her life. For example, Alexis showed some regressed developmental behavior during treatment. Prior to treatment, she slept in her own bed. Post-treatment, she insisted on sleeping in her parents' bed. Alexis created her own coping strategies and participated in a behavior modification program that successfully transitioned her back into her own bed. Alexis created a protection blanket (Figure 4.4) drawn with protection animals to "shield" her from nightmares and a body pillow to replace the presence of her parents. In art therapy, a child achieves mastery when the conflict is expressed, resolved, and integrated (Appleton, 2001). Art therapy was a valuable piece of the comprehensive approach to providing emotional support to Alexis and her family during diagnosis and medical treatment. Today, Alexis continues to benefit from art therapy as she transitions to the survivorship phase of treatment.

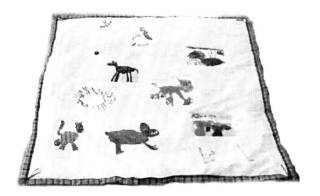

Figure 4.4. *My Protection Blanket,* by Alexis.

Group Art Therapy

The art therapy groups are designed for children who are facing or who have faced medical difficulties. The children find art therapy to be nonverbal, nonthreatening, normal, and fun. The group assists in the sharing of common experiences, the normalization of feelings, and self-expression and self-empowerment.

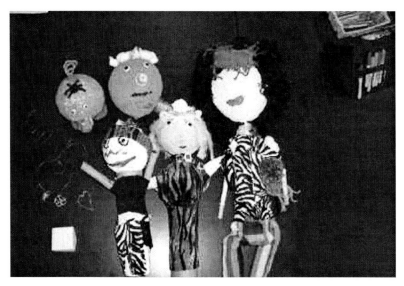

Figure 4.5. *"Me" puppets.*

The art directives include both individual projects and group activities. For example, each child creates a puppet that represents that child
and his or her personality (Figure 4.5). The puppets are used to act out
play scripts the children create on "how to be a good friend." The plays
are videotaped, edited to music, and distributed to the group members.
The activity assists the children in learning coping strategies for transitioning back to school and positive social skills development.

Another art directive is for the group to work together to design their
"ideal hospital" (Figure 4.6). Over several weeks, children in the early
group created their ideal hospital.

Interestingly, the group members included few medical items within
the hospital. Instead, they focused on adding items that would make
their stays more comfortable and enjoyable. For example, they included a hot tub and pool, a disco floor and disco ball, a bowling alley, and
a food court. The children also included thoughtful and insightful items
such as an MRI machine with a television, a timeout chamber for doctors and nurses that the children did not like, teleporters to transport the
doctors quickly to emergencies, and double-sized beds so parents could
stay with them at night. Without prompting, the activity elicited the
sharing of common hospital experiences between group members. In
addition, the group benefited from acting as architects and being able to

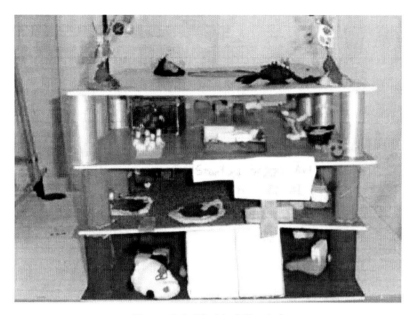

Figure 4.6. *The Ideal Hospital.*

gain some control over the hospital setting. The hospital building created by the early group has become a permanent fixture in the studio. Currently, children in the art therapy group add items and artwork, utilize it for play therapy, and decorate it for the holidays.

Summary

A child with cancer faces many challenges. This chapter explored such children's experiences, challenges, and ways of surviving, both physically and emotionally. It highlighted the emotional effects and psychosocial needs of children with cancer. Cancer survivorship is a lifelong journey and as the rates of survivorship continue to rise, it is vital for children cancer treatment teams to be informed of the struggles their small patients endure. It is important that they understand the support needed to maintain normal development and quality of life. Art therapy is a useful therapeutic technique for working with children, especially children facing illness. Continued research is needed to support and validate the use of art therapy with medical inpatient and outpatient services. The future is bright and the children will continue to offer hope and inspiration for achieving optimal care and success.

References

Appleton, V. (2001). Avenues of hope: Art therapy and the resolution of trauma. *Art Therapy: Journal of the American Art Therapy Association, 18*(1), 6–13.

Bessell, A. (2001). Children surviving cancer: Psychosocial adjustment, quality of life, and school experiences. *The Council for Exceptional Children, 67*(3), 345–359.

Councill, T. (1993). Art therapy with pediatric cancer patients: Helping normal children cope with abnormal circumstances. *Art Therapy: Journal of the American Art Therapy Association, 10*(2), 78–87.

Eiser, C. (2004). *Children with cancer: The quality of life.* Mahwah, NJ: Lawrence Erlbaum.

Erikson, E. (1963). *Childhood and society.* New York: W. W. Norton.

Hodder, H., & Keene, N. (2002). *Childhood cancer: A parent's guide to solid tumor cancers* (2nd ed.). Sebastopol, CA: O'Reilly Media.

Keene, N., Hobbie, W., & Ruccione, K. (2000). *Childhood cancer survivors: A practical guide to your future.* Sebastopol, CA: O'Reilly Media.

Last, B. F., Grootenhuis, M. A., & Eiser, C. (2005). International comparison of psychosocial research on survivors of childhood cancer: Past and future considerations. *Journal of Pediatric Psychology, 30*(1), 99–113.

Leukemia and Lymphoma Society. (2006). *Facts and figures 2005–2006.* Retrieved from http://www.leukemia-lymphoma.org/attachments/National/br_1120235682.pdf

Lusebrink, V. B. (1990). *Imagery and visual expression in therapy.* New York: Plenum.

Malchiodi, C. (Ed.). (1999). *Medical art therapy with children.* London: Jessica Kingsley.

Melman, J., & Sanders, J. (1986). Psychosocial aspects of childhood cancer: A review of the literature. *Journal of Child Psychiatry, 27,* 145–167.

Nainis, N., Paice, J. A., Ratner, J., Wirth, J., Lai, J., & Shott, S. (2006). Relieving symptoms in cancer: Innovative use of art therapy. *Journal of Pain and Symptom Management, 31*(2), 162–169.

National Association of Social Workers & Children's Cause Cancer Advocacy. (2005). *Childhood cancer survivorship: An overview for social workers.* Retrieved from http://www.socialworkers.org/practice/health/cancerFlyer0206.pdf

Patenaude, A. F., & Kupst, M. (2005). Introduction to the special issue: Surviving pediatric cancer: Research gains and goals. *Journal of Pediatric Psychology, 30*(1), 5–8.

Rollins, J. A. (2005). Tell me about it: Drawing as a communication tool for children with cancer. *Journal of Pediatric Oncology Nursing, 22*(4), 203–221.

Ross, D. M., & Ross, S. A. (1984). Stress reduction procedures for the school-age hospitalized leukemic child. *Pediatric Nursing, 10,* 393–395.

Sourkes, B. (1995). *Armfuls of time: The psychological experience of the child with a life-threatening illness.* Pittsburgh, PA: University of Pittsburgh.

Stuyck, K. (2003). *Art therapy helps children affected by cancer express their emotions.* Retrieved from http://arttherapy.wordpress.com/2006/05/28/art-therapy-helps-children-affected-by-cancer/

Sumpter, S. (2005). *Cognitive effects of cancer therapies. Business briefing: U.S. pediatric care.* Retrieved from http://www.touchbriefings.com/pdf/1268/Sumpter.pdf

Teufel, E. (1995). Terminal stage leukemia: Integrating art therapy and family process. *Art Therapy: Journal of the American Art Therapy Association, 12*(1), 51–55.

Chapter 5

FOSTER CARE:
A DEVELOPMENTAL PROBLEM

Carolee Stabno and Sarah Nagle

Dedicated to all of the foster children who have touched our lives.
May they always know how much they matter.

Art, much like the expression of music, is a universal medium that touches each of us. It touches us individually and uniquely, depending upon our experiences, knowledge, and openness to exploration.

Art plays an important role in a child's life, and for a foster child, art plays an even more important role. Because art is language, it helps guide the child's therapeutic journey toward healing and mental health. Children, like adults, have many ways of camouflaging their emotions, and the use of art allows them to enter into a safe zone, a zone where they can explore thoughts, feelings, frustrations, and abuse. Art helps the practitioner understand the underlying thoughts and feelings of the children served.

Some children are removed from the home because they have been neglected, while others may be removed because there is violence in the home or the community as well. Clinical studies of children from violent homes or communities report that "simply witnessing violence or having knowledge of a violent event can have negative implications for children's psychosocial development" (Lewis, Osofsky, & Moore, 1997, p. 278). Drawings, therefore, are used for assessment of the traumas these children may have experienced as well as to encourage the retrieval of traumatic experiences in a safe and distancing way. Studies from South Africa, looking at the impact of violence on preschool children, found that "the more a child is able to express emotional trauma through drawings, the less likely he or she will suffer from PTSD" (Lewis et al., 1997, p. 281). In this chapter, we will share some of our experiences as practitioners with foster children, knowing it will shed some light on the use of art in working with children whose lives have been forever changed by the trauma of separation from their biological families.

General Information about Foster Care

According to the American Academy of Child and Adolescent Psychiatry (2002), more than 500,000 children are currently residing in some form of foster care in the United States, representing a 65 percent increase over the last decade. Half of these children will spend at least two years in the system, and 17 percent of these children will be in the system for five years or more (Badeau & Gesiriech, 2006). Children are placed in the foster care system for a variety of reasons. These reasons include physical, sexual, or emotional abuse, as well as neglect and/or abandonment. Children also enter into the foster care system for specific parental problems. These include physical or mental illness, incarceration, drug or alcohol abuse, AIDS, and death. The goal of foster care is to provide a temporary placement until the child is able to either return home or be adopted. Foster care provides the means to protect these children who need out-of-home care. It is not uncommon, however, for children to return to foster placement because of a failed reunification.

The fastest growing populations in need of foster care are infants and young children, and it is in these early years of life that children experience the critical periods in brain growth and development. Recent research has shown that during this time frame, the brain structures that govern learning processes, personality traits, and the ability to cope with stress and emotions are established and made permanent (Siegel, 2003). If unused, these brain structures will atrophy (American Academy of Pediatrics, 2000). During these critical years, toxic environmental conditions, such as those typically experienced by children in foster placement, can have a negative impact on the child's physical and emotional development. In the first few years of life, physical and mental abuse tends to fix the brain in an acute stress response mode that causes the child to respond in a hypervigilant, fearful manner (Perry & Pollard, 1998). Silver, a pediatric psychologist at The Children's Hospital of Philadelphia, explains that research indicates children who have experienced abuse secrete lower levels of serotonin, a neurotransmitter that influences a child's ability to self-regulate emotions. Increased concentrations of dopamine and testosterone, which are associated with aggression and hypervigilance, have been found in the systems of many of these children. These results cause speculation that when the brain is affected by this imbalance, it reduces the child's capacity for empathy and compassion (Silver, Amster, & Haecker, 1999).

Clearly, children who enter the foster care system bring with them multitudinal issues. Not only are they dealing with phenomenal loss, they are also dealing with the physical and emotional repercussions of abuse, neglect, and/or abandonment inflicted on them by those individuals who were commissioned to care for them—typically, their own parents. As indicated earlier, the child's ability to deal with and heal from these issues is affected by the age of the child at the time of removal from the primary caregiver, the type and length of abuse endured, and the child's emotional attachment to the parental figure(s).

Bowlby (1982) contends that the greatest fear suffered by a child is the threat of abandonment. The foster child is forever plagued with the question, "What is it about me that is so unlovable, so offensive, that my own family could not, and would not, take care of me?" Some foster children find it difficult to feel a sense of permanence or connectedness to their foster families because of their questions and life experiences. What gets added to the mix later is the length of time the child is in placement, the child's own experiences of foster care, and whether or not the child is in a stable placement or moved from home to home.

Removal from Home

What is it like for these children to be removed from their families? What do they have to say about their experiences? Let's begin with discussing their loss.

When a child enters the foster care system, the child is literally removed from all that is familiar. Most children enter foster care with only the clothes they were wearing when they were removed from their families. One little boy, in describing what this experience was like for him, said that it was scary when the police pulled him away from his mother, who was screaming, and put him in the back seat of the police car. But when his dog jumped in the back seat, too, he felt better–until the officer took the dog away from him. He said the officer told him he would see his dog the next day. But that was five years ago, and he hasn't been home since.

When we, as practitioners, think of all the losses these children endure, it's important that we remember the simple things as well. Not only do these children lose their homes, families, neighborhood, friends, schools, favorite foods, clothes, and toys, they also lose that special blanket that used to comfort them when they were scared, or the special teddy with the tattered ears. So how do these children deal with these losses? They talk about them, sometimes verbally, but more often it is through their behavior, their play, and their art that we truly learn how they feel.

Case Studies

JESSE. Jesse, a 4-year-old boy admitted into the foster care system with his baby brother, Mario, became mute immediately after placement. He also became hopelessly sad. Although Jesse was able to engage with members of his foster family through play, he refused to talk to anyone. The only way Jesse communicated was by grunting or pointing at a desired object. If any of the foster family members tried to get him to talk, he would run to another room and cry. Communicating this way wasn't easy for the foster family, but, more importantly, Jesse was in agony. He became overly protective of his little brother, Mario, allowing only his foster mother to hold him. Jesse's refusal to talk also affected Mario, who reacted emotionally. Mario would cry inconsolably when the foster mother left the room, and very often when held, his limbs would be rigid, and his back arched.

During my weekly visits to the home, Jesse would engage with me through nonverbal games. He was beginning to build a strong bond with his foster family, and would excitedly show me things that they had given him, but he would never speak. Week after week, he continued to point and grunt at things he wanted, or wanted me to notice. If Jesse thought I was trying to make him talk, he would run away and engage me in a hide-and-go-seek ritual in the home. About two months later, Jesse once again began his hide-and-go-seek routine with me. This time, however, I turned and went the opposite way, without his knowing, and met him around the corner. We collided in the hallway and sat down next to each other on the floor. As Jesse leaned up against me, I looked across the hall at the mirrored sliding door. I asked Jesse to look in the mirror and said: "See that little boy in the mirror? He looks so very sad." I began naming for him the feelings that I knew he had pent up inside. I began asking questions to the little boy in the mirror. When I asked if that little boy misses his mom, he sat very still, intently looking in the mirror. Within five minutes Jesse began to cry. He was beginning to allow me to reach the injured boy inside. He began to relax and started talking! I asked Jesse to draw how he felt.

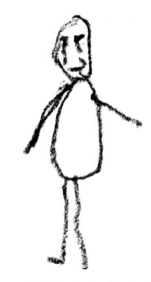

Figure 5.1. *The Crying Boy,* by Jesse, age 5.

During subsequent visits, Jesse talked more and more. His little brother began to calm down as well because Jesse interacted with him in the same way he had prior to placement. Jesse drew many pictures about the sad little boy. Within weeks, he was ready to begin an Early Start Program.

If Jesse had not successfully accomplished Erikson's (1963) first stage of development, learning basic trust versus basic mistrust, he most probably would not have been able to move through his issues of separation and loss, and welcome new exploration and learning. Jesse, however, was able to find his autonomy again and flourish.

BART. Bart, a 14-year-old male, had been in the foster care system four previous times. His mother had serious mental health issues, and was never able to appropriately engage with Bart, who has always been in need of her affection and approval. Instead, during phone calls and sporadic visitations, Bart's mother routinely degraded him, saying very hurtful things, and blaming him for making her life miserable. Although Bart would often hang up on her during phone conversations, asking, "What did I do to deserve this?", he also believed her, and blamed himself for not being able to "fix" his mom. Because of his relationship with his mom, Bart felt shame and guilt. He had trouble sleeping at night, and was extremely anxious. He began to act out, fighting, stealing, running up excessive phone bills, and running away.

Visitations with Mom were minimal. She usually didn't show up for a visit, and when she did, she would spend the time telling Bart he wasn't good enough, or wasn't living up to her expectations. His mother was rageful and explosive. During most of the visits, she would get upset, blame Bart, and charge out the door. After his mother would leave, I would sit with Bart and he would draw. He was accomplished at drawing cartoon and action hero characters. He would make up various creatures and various warriors that often seemed to express how he felt about himself. His warrior monster had a shielded body for protection, and expansive muscles on the torso, legs, and arms. When Bart drew the head, however, it was a simple round circle, which was disconnected from the body at the neck. The eyes were closed, the nose a simple dot, and the mouth a grimace.

While drawing, Bart talked about how much he loved his mom, but said that she had a lot of problems. He said that she always exploded when she was with him and would become very aggressive.

Bart, childlike in many ways, was easy to engage in conversation. He was also like other children; he wanted his mom. At his school he had begun to tell so many stories about himself to other children that he often mixed reality with fantasy, and was unable to separate truth from fiction. Bart was beginning to lose himself in this crucial time of adolescence when his most important task was to develop a sense of self and personal identity.

Bart's art and images were clearly therapeutic, helping him document his early experiences as well as his feelings and emotions about them. He will need to continue in therapy but he has found a way to communicate and work through how trapped he feels inside by his

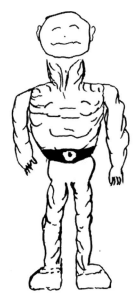

Figure 5.2. *Warrior Monster,* by Bart, age 14.

desire to be loved by his mom, and his knowledge that she will never be there for him.

JASMINE. Jasmine, a five-year-old Caucasian girl, was placed with an African American foster family. When first placed, she was extremely hyperactive and difficult to calm. Prior to placement, Jasmine had been submerged into scalding hot bathwater by her birthmother, and had already undergone several skin grafts. She would need to undergo many more as her body grew and developed. Jasmine's foster family provided her with a very safe, nurturing environment, and she slowly began to calm down and flourish. The foster family consisted of a single mom, her two teenage daughters, and a large extended family that was very tight-knit, yet an open family system. Jasmine fell in love with this family and thrived, not only because she was totally accepted by them, but also because of her own inner strength.

Nurses and doctors were no strangers to Jasmine. When she was taken for doctor visits, she was always surrounded with the support and nurturance of people who cared about her. She stopped hiding her scars and began to feel free enough, and safe enough, to show them.

Jasmine's foster family encouraged many experiential activities, which she loved. She became more even-tempered and better able to regulate her emotional responses. She no longer had severe meltdowns or tantrums. Despite her deformities, she engaged well with other children her age, as well as with adults. Jasmine was able to establish close, loving attachments to her foster family, as was evidenced in weekly therapeutic visits to the home. Jasmine had her own painting easel, and drawing and finger-painting became strong tools of expression for her. After a year in placement, this family adopted Jasmine. She gained not only a family, but also a family who was in tune with this traumatized child, and her need for self-expression and exploration. As Jasmine grew over the years, she did need more skin grafts, and she continued to use art as a way to make sense of the world and to express her feelings.

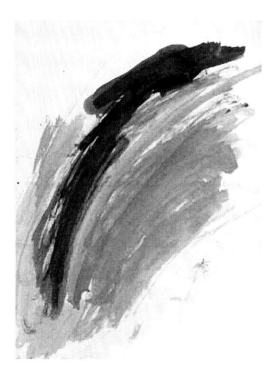

Figure 5.3. *A Rainbow*, by Jasmine, (early in placement).

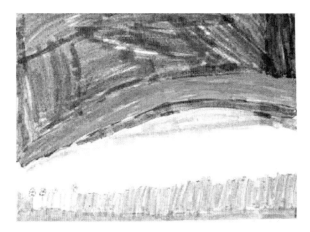

Figure 5.4. *A Rainbow,* by Jasmine, (3 months after placement).

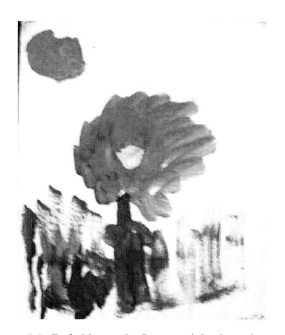

Figure 5.5. *Early Morning,* by Jasmine, (after her adoption).

DERALLY. Derally was a 15-year-old Samoan girl who came into the foster care system in her third month of pregnancy. She had a severe sexual abuse history, and had undergone one, if not two, abortions prior to placement. She came into placement with a diagnosis of post-traumatic stress disorder and depression. She had significant delays in learning, as did her mother and her grandmother. After having her baby, Allison, Derally stayed with her child in a special foster care program that would have enabled her to graduate from high school and learn life tools before she was emancipated. Unfortunately, when she was 18 years old, the school reported that Derally's vocational test results were too low to put her into a vocational program. She was then told that her scores were too high to qualify for the help of the local regional center. At this point, the county was not able to provide, or was not aware of, resources that could help Derally transition from foster care to adulthood, with a baby, into the community.

During this time of chaos, Derally took two-year-old Ali to a party, and while at the party, one of the girls let the baby drink from her wine cooler. One of the other girls at the party reported the incident to Child Protective Services, and although there were no other incidents, Derally lost her baby to the dependency of the court. She was told that she was unable to make the right choices for her child, and therefore couldn't keep her. Derally was a true victim of society. She didn't qualify for services that would help her make the right choices, nor did she have the skills to help her fight for her rights in court. The baby was adopted within one year, and Derally's world fell apart. To be expected, Derally soon became pregnant again, and within her first trimester, had a miscarriage. Shortly thereafter, the county sent Derally back to live with her mother, saying that she was uncooperative. Derally's therapist, a licensed psychologist and board certified art therapist, worked with her during her placement in foster care, particularly focusing on good memories she had shared with her daughter and the dreams she had for the future.

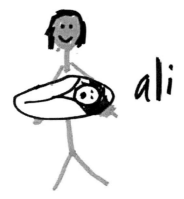

Figure 5.6 *Alison's birth,* by Derally.

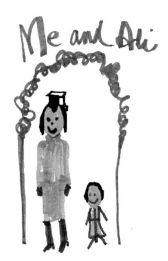
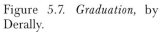

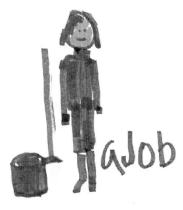

Figure 5.8. *My future job at Marine World*, by Derally.

Figure 5.7. *Graduation*, by Derally.

Postscript. Within three years of being sent home, Derally had two children, one of whom is developmentally delayed. She continues to live with her mother and has no prospect for a life different than what she has always known. She has long since given up on getting a job, having grown up in a home that relied on the welfare system for survival. Would Derally's life be different than it is today if there had been appropriate services available for a young person whose IQ was too low for vocational training, and too high to qualify for regional center services? How many youth are there like Derally, who never had adequate parenting and literally fall through the cracks of social care as they try to go out on their own?

Continuing Challenges

In the United States today there is a genuine need for foster care, and when it works, it is exceptional and family and child are fortunate. But foster care is a developmental issue. Once a child is removed from his or her home, no matter how dysfunctional, and goes into the system, that child's life is forever changed, as we have seen above. There are many times, however, when foster care doesn't work, foster parents burn out, and children are moved from placement to placement, or reunified too quickly, only to have the reunification fail. Youth in foster care often move into adulthood without having developed relational support, skills, or experience.

Foster Parent Perspective

So what are the experiences of foster parents and foster families? Being a foster parent has its joys, but it also has its pitfalls. A foster parent must tolerate case managers, social workers, therapists, and attorneys entering the home on a regular basis, often unannounced. Further, it is often difficult for foster parents to understand why a child would still love, and long for, the mother who severely abused him or her, particularly when the foster parents are providing the child with safety, love, and security, perhaps the first the child has ever known. If foster parents think that a foster child will show gratitude for being taken in and given a home, they need to think again.

In this chapter, we've talked about losses from the foster child's perspective, but what about the losses a foster parent endures? Foster parents bring a child into their home, providing the child with love, nurturance, and support. Eventually they develop a strong, loving attachment with this child, who will then, more than likely, leave within one or two years. The finality of these goodbyes is often very, very painful, particularly when they are endured by foster parents over and over again.

Youth in Foster Care

Most foster youth become homeless or are incarcerated shortly after they emancipate into adulthood. Further, less than nine percent ever receive college degrees (Jacobs, 2006). Those of us who work in foster care are aware that additional transitional services and training are needed for most youth in foster care moving into adulthood if we want them to succeed in independent living in adulthood.

The significance of this problem has been recognized by Howard Jacobs (2006), Director of Public Affairs and Government Relations, G.L.A.S.S. Jacobs believes that the way foster care advocates communicate with and respect one another's roles needs the most change. He argues that foster children, and former foster children, are not listened to by county administrators or adult advocates, and notes that what foster youth think about services is generally considered to be irrelevant. Until child advocates, including attorneys, judges, and government administrators, listen to the voices of youth and their service providers, real, substantive change will not occur. "The system will remain chaotic, as youth with greater needs end up in out-of-home care" (Jacobs, 2006, p. 6).

Further complicating emancipation is the actual developmental stage at which this process begins and ends: adolescence. Adolescence is, by nature, a chaotic time. It is a normal developmental issue. The teen is beginning to form his or her own identity, and in order to do this successfully, the teen begins to resist parental rules (see Chapter 7, Adolescents, Identity, Addiction, and Images, and Chapter 9, The Deviant Adolescent). This is difficult enough for the birth parent to experience, but when a foster parent experiences it, it can be daunting, daunting because the system has rules, and these rules are often incompatible with the teen's developmental task of separation/individuation. The adolescent foster child ready for more independence is not allowed to be left home alone at any time, and not allowed to have a key to the house (because, of course, the foster child cannot be in the home alone). To complicate matters further, in adolescence foster children begin to more fully understand all they have lost. The grief they feel over these losses often results in destructive behaviors such as drinking, drugs, fighting, etc. According to Erikson (1963), the adolescent's basic conflict is identity vs. role confusion. The very nature of foster care places a child in an "identity vs. role confusion" state. A foster child may rightfully wonder, "Who am I, really? Am I like my foster dad, who is a successful engineer, or am I like my birthfather, who is in prison for life?" It is during this critical developmental stage that the foster child ages out of the system, and is left to fend for him or herself.

State and federal policies regulate the age at which a foster child must leave the child welfare system, which is currently 18 years of age. States vary widely in the services they offer to foster children over the age of 18. An 18-year-old, however, is still an adolescent. And an 18-year-old foster child is an adolescent with incredibly difficult issues with which to contend. Where, and with whom, will these teens be able to connect as young adults, given the harsh demands of society? Who will be their guide?

Most young people make a safe passage from adolescence to adulthood with the support of their families, other caring adults, communities, and schools. Foster children, however, have few supports. They need help to find the right paths where they can succeed.

Conclusion

There is, however, exciting new hope for these youth, and it's because of a program called "Connected by 25." Simply stated, this program is designed to help foster children who "age out" of the system to make successful transitions to adulthood. This program is funded by local and national foundations, and tries to connect these vulnerable young people to education, housing, employment, banks, and support systems by the age of 25. It focuses on economic success because the ability to support oneself and accumulate assets often predicts future success in life. For this new program to be successful, however, it is imperative that the services provided meet the foster child at his or her own developmental level–which may or may not be the level one might expect of an average 18-year-old.

As demonstrated in this chapter, formulating a treatment plan for a foster child isn't linear, it's multifaceted. It includes knowledge of child development, and the developmental level of the child during the trauma and subsequent removal from home. It includes remembering that the key to minimizing the long-term effects of traumatic events on the child's brain is early intervention. For children and youth, this means right-hemisphere interventions that tap into the feelings they never learned. It includes specific emphasis on separation, attachment, and relationship-based interventions, and knowledge of the biological bases of behavior. Successful treatment requires a safe place to explore the traumas of childhood, and a safe place to explore the challenging behaviors that develop over time as a result of the traumas. Successful treatment often occurs without words.

References

American Academy of Child and Adolescent Psychiatry. (2002, January). *Facts for families: Foster care.* Retrieved April 28, 2006, from http://www.aacap.org/publications/factsfam/64.htm

American Academy of Pediatrics, Committee on Early Childhood, Adoption and Dependent Care. (2000, November). Developmental issues for young children in foster care. *Early Childhood Newsletter, 106*(5), 1145–1150. Retrieved April 28,

2006, from http://aappolicy.aappublications.org/cgi/content/full/pediatrics;106/5/1145

American Academy of Pediatrics, Committee on Early Childhood, Adoption, and Dependent Care. (2002, March). Improving mental health outcomes for young children in foster care. *Early Childhood Newsletter.* Retrieved July 2, 2006, from www.aappolicy.aappublicaions.org/cgi/content/full/pediatrics;109/3/536

Badeau, S., & Gesiriech, S. (2006). A child's journey through the child welfare system. *The Pew Commission on Children in Foster Care.* Retrieved September 22, 2006, from http://pewfostercare.org/docs/index.php?DocID=24

Bowlby, J. (1982). *Attachment and loss. Vol. 1: Attachment.* (2nd ed). New York: Basic Books.

Erikson, E. (1963). *Childhood and society* (2nd ed.). New York: W. W. Norton.

Jacobs, H. (2006, June). Foster Care vs HIV. Better outcomes with less money. National Association of Social Workers. *California News. (32)*9.

Lewis, M., Osofsky, J., & Moore, M. (1997). Violent Cities, violent streets: Children draw their neighborhoods. In I. J. Osofsky (Ed.), *Children in a Violent Society* (pp. 277–322). New York: Guilford Press.

Perry, P., & Pollard, R. (1998). Homeostasis, stress, trauma and adoption: A neurodevelopmental view of childhood trauma. *Child & Adolescent Psychiatric Clinics of North America, 7*(1), 33–51.

Siegel, D. (2003). An interpersonal neurobiology of psychotherapy: The developing mind and the resolution of trauma. In M. Soloman & D. Siegel (Eds.), *Healing Trauma: Attachment, mind, body, and brain* (pp. 1–56). New York: W. W. Norton.

Silver, J. A., Amster, B. J., & Haecker, T. (1999). *Young children in foster care: A guide for professionals.* Baltimore: Paul H. Brookes.

Chapter 6

THE MAGIC HOUR: SUCCESS WITH DIFFICULT CHILDREN

Roberta Hauser and DeAnn Acton

Dedicated to our children, Neil and Caya, who help us stay balanced.

Introduction

"Throughout the industrialized world, as well as in most developing areas, the years of middle childhood are devoted to education. . . . The first day of school is considered one of the most important transition points in a child's life" (Bee & Boyd, 2003, p. 217). The child moves from being a preschooler into a personal and cultural learning experience as a "big kid." Parents mark the day in many ways. They provide new school supplies and clothes. They take pictures of the children with friends, on the school bus, or in their classrooms. For some children, however, for those who will exhibit or have exhibited problem behaviors in and outside of the classroom, for those who receive negative responses from their classmates and adults, for those who will be or those already labeled by teachers, counselors, school districts, and even parents, this day begins tentatively with caution and even fear. For these children, this may not be the beginning of Erikson's fourth developmental stage, industry. Instead, the child may spiral into the alternative stage, developing a deep feeling of inferiority.

How can this tragic experience be curtailed? Understanding the four major contributing factors (biological, familial, cultural, and school-related) is helpful in understanding the ways that behavior problems can be remediated (Anderson, 1992). This chapter will focus on the success of treating these children in art therapy groups run through a county mental health program in collaboration with the county's school of education. It will be a summary of what the two authors have experienced working for over 25 years in psychiatric hospitals, day treatment centers, and special education school settings.

The Magic Hour

Six little boys sit eagerly around a rectangular table. They are excited and finding it difficult to wait patiently. For many of the children, this is their favorite hour of the day. Language and reading deficits and other learning differences can be momentarily set aside. Here, their inexhaustible energy and anxious emotions are contained within the boundaries of one hour, in which they are creating a single art project. The children's eyes brighten as they look at the example provided by the art therapist, and although they feel some uncertainty around whether or not they can succeed, they all can't wait to try.

Throughout the United States, art therapy groups have long been a staple of classrooms with difficult children (Arrington, 1979). These groups allow children a place to use their right-hemisphere communication patterns for expression, hands-on skills building, and for repairing a sometimes much-damaged sense of self (Liebmann, 1986).

Example: Jack. Jack, age 10, was pretty angry. This was his third classroom this year. He had been removed from his initial classroom because of disruptive behaviors and fighting. When the police had been called to the school three times in one week, the principal felt that Jack would be better served in a different setting. He was then transferred to a special classroom for emotionally disturbed youngsters. His anger escalated. This time, it was decided that Jack needed more structure and additional adult supervision. He was transferred to a milieu classroom in a different setting run by the county school district. At the same time, Jack disclosed to a teacher that he was being abused at home, and he was moved out of the only home he had ever known into foster care. Issues of loss and anxiety were overwhelming. Depression and anxiety exacerbated Jack's already acute learning disabilities.

Art Therapy Group Model

The art therapy group serves as a model community, where each member must learn how to act appropriately, share, and withhold judgment. The groups are also useful as a training ground for developing improved interpersonal skills (Anderson, 1992; Rubin, 1978).

These clients, whom we will refer to as "kids," are children that for many years have had repeated negative experiences in school. These school failures, changes, and disruptions, starting in the early grades, have caused significant damage to self-esteem and motivation. These kids, a majority of them boys, no longer approach school with curiosity or a "love for learning." Will they miss Erikson's (1963) industry stage, falling instead into the abyss of inferiority?

These kids come to school with their guard up, defending against being exposed or humiliated. They fear that someone may discover that they cannot read or sit still for five minutes. They can't spell or add or subtract in a simple math problem. They arrive at school burdened, defended, anxious, isolated, defeated, and, sadly, in a state of fear. This fear is presented in many ways, such as depression, grouchiness, rudeness, aggressiveness, hostility, humor, arrogance, anxiety, and even a sort of insidious chronic pessimism. The most common diagnoses listed in the *Diagnostic and Statistical Manual of Mental Disorders-IV-TR* (APA, 2000) found in concert with learning disabilities are depression, dysthymia, conduct disorder, intermittent explosive disorder, attention deficit disorders, obsessive compulsive disorder, reactive attachment disorder, and anxiety disorders.

These kids are generally distrustful of adults. Relationship building is a slow and tenuous process that takes patience and a firm, consistent adult. Most of these kids feel defeated, tired of failing, and unwilling to make even an attempt at a new experience. Self-deprecating remarks and insulting attacks on the intelligence of others are common. Generally, these kids are emotionally immature for their chronological age and quick to regress further when pushed or challenged. These are children with fragile self-esteem who need a continuous flow of positive feedback in any environment where they are exploring something new or different.

Most special education students have been moved away from their original school peers in regular education, maybe across the campus or sometimes across the county. They are initially socially isolated and put in with special education students of mixed ages with a variety of problems. They are asked to start over every time they are moved from one class setting to another, which increases their distrustfulness and isolation. As a group, they are painfully socially awkward. Because they are used to classes that are homogenous by grade, the new classrooms can feel alienating. In a regular education classroom, children often move from one classroom to the next within any particular day. They meet with a diversity of learning opportunities, students, and teachers. In the special education classroom, students are often with the same teacher and students for the entire school day for years at a time. This can be a safer, more appropriate learning situation, but it is also a huge social challenge, when every regular education middle school kid is already struggling socially.

The behavior-disordered student faces initial rejections and failures, loss of social group and school, loss of self-esteem around school performance, increased tension in family relationships, and an increased pressure to improve or perform. The behavior-disordered child needs advocacy. Such children need parents to help them initially to identify their disorders, get the right assessments, activate the school system to respond to their newly identified disorders or emotional problems, and provide the best educational setting possible for these children. As many parents try to cope on a daily basis with their own issues, their special-education children may have no one to advocate on their behalf, and ultimately may be ignored by the larger school system. Financial necessity may require that some family members have two or three jobs. Students may have no one at home to help with homework, reinforce learning, or recognize when they are having difficulty within the school system. Or, even worse, many children have family members whose own mental health issues or substance addictions create a chaotic home environment where the child's needs for safety and advocacy can never be met. Family therapy, offered as a means of helping to work through those issues, may often be unused.

Goals

There are three goals that are specific to this population. They are (1) to regulate the child's negative affect, (2) to improve his sense of self, and (3) to provide a safe environment where he and other participants can make friends.

The first goal, helping the children self-regulate negative affect so they are able to focus on tasks and complete assignments, is well-suited to the art therapy group. Here, the children understand that through the behavior management system employed in all other groups, negative behaviors will be consequenced. In the children's excitement to complete their art projects, they are more able to attend to directions and limits in order to express themselves and still have something very special that they can take home at the end of the day. As the children become more comfortable within the art group, they take more risks and are better able to handle the frustration connected with more difficult projects. They also begin to recognize that the simple making of art feels good and later they are able to use this skill outside of the art group to de-escalate when they are feeling overwhelmed by negative emotions.

A second goal is to improve the child's overall sense of self through improved feelings of competency. As the children learn how to use the diverse tools presented to them and to complete projects of which they are proud, their sense of proficiency increases. When these pieces are later displayed in the classroom or in an art show, these positive feelings of self are amplified. When a child takes his or her artwork home, it is a positive communication from the school to the family. When a child's art work is exhibited at school, it is a positive communication to the child.

A third goal is to give the children a safe environment where they can improve those skills necessary to both make and keep friends. Learning how to share art supplies and space, to listen to the group facilitator and their peers, to give and receive positive feedback, and to be appropriate within the context of the art group can be translated into healthier relationships in the classroom and in their communities.

Example: Jack. It was Jack's second time-out. He had received warnings earlier for speaking out of turn. When he called a peer a name, he received his first time-out. Jack returned to the group, only to continue the insults. He was asked to go back to his desk. Jack was angry and yelled from across the room. He was advised that if he was not able to control his behavior, he would be asked to sit outside of the door of the classroom. Jack became quiet. His anger turned to sadness. He pleaded to be let back into group. He wanted to finish his project. He didn't like the idea of the other children finishing without him.

Making Art

Making art can be relaxing and inherently healing through its ability to allow for the creative and sometimes spontaneous expression of its participants (Anderson, 1992). Art can also be provocative. The sensory materials can elicit regressive tendencies and at times the spontaneous nature of art making can trigger traumatic thoughts that were previously buried. In a group where children are learning basic social skills, group dynamics create another layer of possible stress. Many art therapists have learned through painful experience that they must find ways to combine the role of limit-setter and consequence-giver with that of nurturer and healer. A consistent structure with clear limits and expectations and a means for positive reinforcement distinguishes the successful art therapy group from pandemonium.

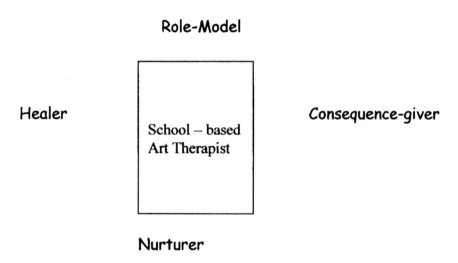

Figure 6.1. Various roles of the school-based art therapist.

Group Rules

The "group rules" are simple. They allow each participant to have a basic understanding of what is expected and what behaviors will be unacceptable within the context of the group. If there are too many rules, the group will become a daunting place where there is no room for safe exploration. If the art therapist makes the mistake of creating a rule to apply to every negative behavior she thinks of, then something will be forgotten and classroom participants will find the loopholes.

Art therapy groups have four basic rules:

1. Be safe!
2. Follow directions.

3. Be respectful.
4. Ask permission.

Although there are only four group rules, they cover a myriad of negative behaviors without having to list each of them. When the rules are first introduced to the group, students are asked to help explain what behaviors might fit under each rule. The first rule, "Be safe," covers everything from using art materials properly to students keeping their hands and feet to themselves. The second rule, "Follow directions," covers listening to group leaders and doing the art process. The third rule, "Be respectful," includes sharing materials, being nonjudgmental, and not interrupting. The fourth and last rule, "Ask permission," requires that students ask permission to get out of their seats as well as to use particular materials.

Group Structure

Aside from clear rules, a successful art group also needs structure. Many of the students in art therapy groups come from chaotic and often unpredictable environments. Family members come and go. It is not unusual for children to be enrolled in three or four schools in one year. The art therapy group creates a structure through a consistent schedule of events, the presentation of materials, a collaborative relationship with school staff, and time management.

Each art therapy group begins and ends in the same way each week. The group begins with a reading aloud of the group rules by group participants. The group ends with each participant answering a process question posed by the facilitator. These opening and closing rituals act as a container and help each student transition in and out of the group process. Between the opening and closing rituals is the presentation of the art project. Because the students in art therapy groups are often severely learning disabled, it is important to present each project in clear and concise steps. These steps must be given one or two at a time. When working with learning disabled populations, giving any more than two steps at a time can overwhelm and create confusion for the participants. An example of a completed art project proves beneficial in motivating the students to attempt the project and in helping them to understand the expectations.

A second way of creating structure in the art therapy group centers on the presentation of art materials. Issues of scarcity and competitiveness are often triggered when the art supplies are presented during the onset of group. The children often have internal questions such as, "Will she have enough for me?" or "Will I get the materials I want?" These internal questions suggest the students' own struggles outside of the art group to get their basic needs met. Providing the students with adequate and well-organized materials assists in group structure. Eliminating unnecessary art materials from the table as soon as they have been used helps to create space and minimize clutter and distractions.

Group structure is maintained through successful collaboration with the classroom staff. The art therapy group is organized to fit into the overall structure of the classroom. At home, children become acutely aware when parents are not aligned or have different expectations. This is also true of the educational team. It is important that the art therapy group not mimic this dysfunctional pattern when working with children. Classroom staff should continue to give individual support to students and to be part of the setting of limits. Use of a consistent vocabulary helps children understand that the art therapist and staff form a cohesive unit. If the word "warning" is used to alert a student when he is losing points or is about to receive a time-out, all staff must use this same word. Using a different term, such as "chance," serves to confuse the student. A successful collaboration also utilizes the knowledge and experience of both the art therapist and the classroom staff. Briefings between educators and therapist about a child's current behavioral status assist each in predicting difficult behaviors and establishing systems to curtail those behaviors if they appear in the group.

Group structure is also created through time management skills. Many of these children reside in homes where life is never consistent. They often cannot predict a caretaker's mood, when they will receive dinner, or an often-absent parent's appearance in the home. All of this unpredictability creates anxiety. Beginning and ending each group at a consistent time helps to create a special container for each child's experience within the group. For insecure children, transitions are difficult. For disorganized students who might worry about completing a project, letting them know that their time is up without fair warning can create complications that last far after the art therapist leaves the classroom. Giving 15-, 10-, and 5-minute warnings creates safety in the group and helps each student learn how to transition effectively from one task to another. It also helps them practice being in control of some of their own time.

Aside from providing clear expectations and a solid structure, the art therapist also motivates positive behaviors in the group. Time spent in the art therapy group is frequently monitored by classroom staff and included in the classroom point system. Therefore, it is important for the art therapist to provide means for motivating students. For some children, positive feedback regarding their behavior and projects is all that is needed to keep negative behaviors in check. Other children find intrinsic motivation from a completed project of which they are proud.

Unfortunately, there must also be a system to consequence negative behaviors. In art therapy groups, the time-out has been the most effective means of controlling negative acting-out behaviors and keeping the group safe. When given a time-out, the student is asked to go to his or her desk, remain quiet, and wait for an adult to ask him or her back into the group. If the student continues to need several time-outs in a short period of time, he or she may be asked to complete the art project at his or her desk. Because each child is aware of the expectations for the group, a time-out generally does not come as a surprise. Testing the limits and the limit setter is an important task for many children. Questions such as "Can you keep me safe?" or "Will you do what you say?" are answered by how well you can hold children accountable for their behaviors. Time-outs are most effective when the limit setter has a flat affect, expects compliance, and verbalizes positive outcomes for following directions.

When creating a clear classroom structure, understanding group process is important (Yalom, 1975). Each group moves through a pattern of behaviors in order to both create identity and solidify its purpose. Each phase of group development comes with different needs and tasks. Knowing which phase of group the art therapy group is currently experiencing helps the therapist to create appropriate interventions and questions. An experienced group leader is aware that these phases may not always be sequential. A group can move through one stage only to regress to a previous stage of development. Groups can become stuck in any one stage and may need the art therapist to help them move forward.

The following charts are included to assist the reader. Chart A describes different phases of groups, the tasks associated with each phase, and art materials and projects appropriate for each phase. Chart B includes information on how best to support a group in moving through each phase and information regarding process questions.

Process questions are utilized to consciously connect the phases of group to each group member. When a group is struggling to understand rules and structure, questions of safety become important. When a group is saying goodbye, questions that seek to acknowledge group members' contributions are both necessary and validating.

Tool Chest

The following guidelines are important when working with behavior-disordered and learning-disabled children. References and suggestions for working with difficult children are included in what we refer to as the **Tool Chest.**

- Set clear rules and expectations and post them on the wall!
- Work as a part of a team.
- Create situations where a child can feel successful.
- Provide examples of art directives as another means of explanation.
- Understand your population and know their ability levels.
- Reduce distractions.
- Provide both clear verbal directions and a visual demonstration.
- Provide projects that can be completed in the allotted time.
- Recognize the signs of frustration and intervene proactively.
- Expect resistance and plan for it.
- Avoid humiliating students. Avoid public feedback.
- Don't respond negatively to copying. Copying can be an effective means of coping.
- Use at least three directives with each project to extend the attention span and the learning process.
- Encourage flexibility in problem solving. Be aware of words like "perfect."
- Manage time effectively and help clients become aware of time.
- Provide encouragement!

An Art Show

An art show is a great acknowledgement of a student's creative work. If a treatment setting is one where an art show is appropriate, taking into consideration issues of confidentiality and client needs, it can be a powerful experience for both student and therapist alike. An art show expands a student's self-expression and safely shares it with an appreciative audience. It reinforces the value of self-expression and the students begin to see themselves with new identities and labels, as artists. The art show includes family members as part of the experience. Students are able to share the work that they have done and raise feelings of competency.

A child placed in mainstream education will often receive many opportunities for positive public praise. Children join sports teams, learn how to dance, participate in school plays, or are able to attend awards ceremonies where family and friends share in their accomplishments. Many behavior-disordered students, however, do not have these same opportunities. Because of its more passive nature, an art show is a safe way to engage public support and normalcy for these students with special needs. The student's work is framed, titled, and presented, emphasizing its importance to the student, family, and community. Awards and certificates are given to each participant to further acknowledge his or her capability and cooperation in the art show.

An art exhibition has a secondary benefit of helping others within a treatment team to look at a student differently. Staff and parents begin to understand the important role that art plays for each student. They also may begin to see strengths that they had not seen before. The artwork is often placed in a public space within a school, and is therefore shared with others within a student community who may not have direct contact with a particular student.

An art exhibit held at the end of a school year has the additional benefit of providing closure for the students. It serves as a celebration, acknowledging everyone's work and participation. Art is a symbol of the self. An art show further validates the importance and beauty of each of the participants.

Example: Jack. The walls are covered in a diverse array of artwork. Months of work have culminated into this final display of color and hard work. Jack enters the room with his foster parents. His eyes search the walls immediately. One of the therapists notices Jack's anxious looks and leads him to the wall where his artwork hangs. Beside his artwork is his name. Jack looks at his painting and begins to smile. He shows his foster family, who share his excitement in seeing his name and the artwork that he created.

Appendix A
Stages of Group–Focus and Projects

Phase	Tasks/Focus of Group	Art Materials/Projects
Phase 1 **Coming Together** (2–3 weeks)	Joining Why are we here? Who are you? Who am I? What's the group about? What are the rules?	Very easy to use Simple projects Quick success Low expectations
Phase 2 **Finding the Limits** (1–3 months)	Who is in charge? What are our group goals? What are our individual goals? What are the rules? What are the consequences? What are the rewards?	Simple materials Not a lot of chaos Therapist chooses projects No fluid materials Take a group photo
Phase 3 **Becoming a Group** (1–2 months)	Establish group cohesion Sticking to the routine Consistency in structure Rules = safety How do we make a group decision?	Projects with more steps Increase difficulty Begin working in dyads Cooperative projects **Take photos**
Phase 4 **Working Together** (1–2 months)	Trust is established Sense of comfort Group decision making Client leadership	Increasingly complex tasks and materials Group projects Project that take 2–3 sessions Projects directly related to issues **Take photos**
Phase 5 **Saying Goodbye** (1 month–6 weeks)	Goals What did we accomplish? Identify low points and high points. Honor each other in some way. Create opportunities to acknowledge and aware each group member. Elicit positive future optimism.	Create transitional objects. Create photo albums, autograph books, and group books. Go back to individual projects. Create a gift of artwork. Produce an art show of student Work.

Appendix B
Stages of Group–Support and Process

Phase	Level of Support	Process Content "Question of the day"
Phase 1 **Coming Together** (2–3 weeks)	Use examples. Write steps clearly on the board. Strong limit setting. Offer lots of help. Demonstrate the materials.	Questions are orientation, joining, superficial, and nonconfrontational. "Why are we here?"
Phase 2 **Finding the Limits** (1–3 months)	Same level of support as in the forming stage, with strong limit setting emphasized by the therapist. Repeat directions. Earn rewards quickly.	Questions around evaluation, safety, trust. Questions to establish the routine of the group. Watch for issues around "pecking order" and how well the group fits together.
Phase 3 **Becoming a Group** (1–2 months)	Move towards less help. Show examples of project and put away. Manage the materials.	Questions investigating how we are the same and different. Decreasing acting out behaviors. Evaluating how deeply the group will be able to go into their presenting issues. Questions to reduce defensiveness.
Phase 4 **Working Together** (1–2 months)	Client may lead group. More independent work. Clients do the work. Clients make more choices. Therapist can step back if group is functioning well. Longer time to earn rewards.	How do you function in group? What is your issue? Can you share it? What is it like to be in the group? Questions that connect art with issues.
Phase 5 **Saying Goodbye** (1 months–6 weeks)	Therapist moves back into the lead. Safety around emotional expression. Appropriate good-byes. What have you earned? Cash out points.	Who has been here? Acknowledge everyone. Honest feedback. Address good-bye and loss issues. How did relationships in the group help you? Or not?

Appendix C
Suggested Project Ideas and Directions for Art Therapist

Phase	Project	Preparation Work & Materials	Directions	Process Question	Goal
Phase 1 **Coming Together** (2–3 weeks)	**Name Banner**	• Cut out banners and provide a completed example of project possibilities: Banners. • Provide Paper and Markers	• Demonstrate to client how he or she can draw his or her name in creative letters and create an artistic background using markers.	• Share one thing about your name. • Share one thing you observed today.	• Become familiar with each other
Phase 2 **Finding the Limits** (1–3 months)	**Personal Car**	• Cut car shapes out of poster board. • Share examples of cars. • Provide paper, markers and glue.	• Demonstrate to client how he or she can design his or her own car using markers, or colored paper on car-shaped paper provided.	• Who is in the car? • Whose car is it? • Where is it going? • Where would you like to go in it?	• Become familiar with each other • Become comfortable with art supplies
	Leather Pouch	• Share completed examples of leather pouches. • Provide leather and tools for projects.	• Demonstrate to client how to use leather tools and create a pouch. • Assist clients in choosing a color and leather for laces and a pouch.	• What can it hold? • How would someone know it was yours?	• Move away from drawing • Connect clients to their work

(continues)

Phase	Project	Preparation Work & Materials	Directions	Process Question	Goal
Phase 3 **Becoming a Group** (1–2 months)	**Clay Head**	• Share completed examples of clay projects. • Instruct clients as to how to work with clay. • Provide clay and clay tools.	• Demonstrate to clients how to work with clay and keep it moist. Ask group members to follow the leader in clay exercises and then work on their individual projects. • Provide examples of people, animals, and monsters. • Assist clients in creating their own original heads.	• Does your head have a name? What is it? • How did you make your decisions along the way?	• Introduce new materials • Connect clients to their work
	Feeling Faces	• Cut out masks so that machine tape can slide through eyes and mouth area. • Masks & markers • Machine tape	• Demonstrate how tape can change the expression on a premade mask by pulling tape through the eye and mouth openings.	• What feelings does your mask express? • What feelings are difficult for you?	• Emotion awareness • Self-exploration
Phase 4 **Working Together** (1–2 months)	**Personal Shields**	• Cut out large shields for each group member. • Assist clients in collecting symbols. • Provide shields, symbols, markers, pencils	• Demonstrate how each client can create a personal shield by selecting symbols that relate to interests and culture. • Provide clients with examples of symbols from many differing cultures.	• How does the shield represent you? • What would you like to share about your shield? • What are its positive qualities?	• Direct personal expression and ownership

Making a Home	• Provide a variety of small animals for clients to select (birds, animals or fish). • Provide markers and a variety of paper materials.	• Demonstrate to each client how to use paper and natural materials to create a home and an environment for their animal. • Ask each client to select and share three adjectives describing his or her animal. • Ask each client to select and share three objectives describing the home they created for his or her animal.	• What adjectives did you choose? • Why?	• Look at strengths of client • Look at defenses of client • Look for cooping strategies of client

(continues)

Phase	Project	Preparation Work & Materials	Directions	Process Question	Goal
Phase 5 **Saying Goodbye** (1 months–6 weeks)	**Goodbye Album and Art Show of student work if appropriate.**	• Provide some completed examples of Goodbye albums. • Provide a variety of ribbon and paper. • Include photos of group members both individually and as part of the group. • Help students select pictures and mats for the art show. • Let them assist in hanging the show and creating a Show Brochure.	• Ask each client to make an album dealing with saying goodbye. • Demonstrate to each client how to make a cover for their album using photos, collage materials or drawings. • Assist group members in making an album page for every other group member, Include drawings, autographs, poems, and personal memories. • Assist members in exchanging the memory pages they have made for fellow group members. • Bind the album.	• What have you accomplished in the group? • What has the group accomplished? • What does the future look like? • What changes have you made? • What have the relationships in the group meant to you?	• Provide closure and a transitional object • Ask clients to draw a positive frame around a painful experience

Appendix D
Examples of Project Ideas

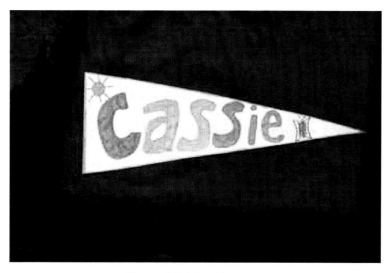

Figure 6.2. Name banner.

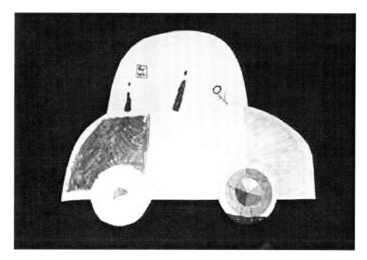

Figure 6.3. Personal car.

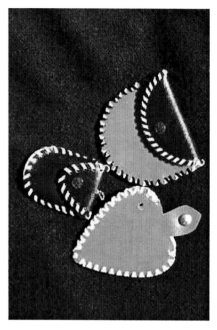

Figure 6.4. Leather pouch.

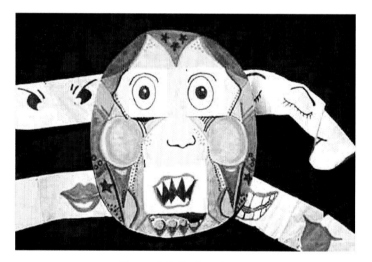

Figure 6.5. Feeling faces.

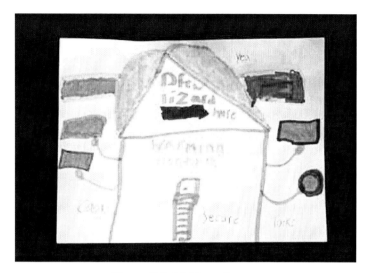

Figure 6.6. Making a home.

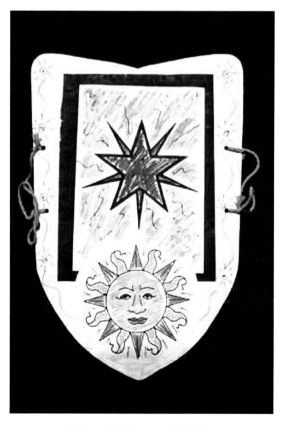

Figure 6.7. Personal shields.

References

American Psychiatric Association. (1994). *Diagnostic and Statistical Manual of Mental Disorders* (4th ed.). Washington, DC: Author.

Anderson, F. (1992). *Art for all the children: Approaches to art therapy for children with disabilities*. Springfield, IL: Charles C Thomas.

Arrington, D. (1979). Art rapp: Innovative use of art therapy in public schools. *Proceedings of the Tenth Annual Conference of The American Art Therapy Association,* Los Angeles, CA, 37–39.

Bee, H., & Boyd, D. (2003). *Lifespan development* (3rd ed.). Boston: Allan and Bacon.

Erikson, E. (1963). *Childhood and society* (2nd ed.). New York: W. W. Norton.

Liebmann, M. (1986). *Art therapy for groups: A handbook of themes, games and exercises*. Cambridge, MA: Brookline Books.

Rubin, J. (1978). *Child art therapy: Understanding and helping children grow through art*. New York: Van Nostrand Reinhold.

Yalom, I. D. (1975). *The theory and practice of group psychotherapy*. New York: Basic Books.

Chapter 7

ADOLESCENTS, IDENTITY, ADDICTION, AND IMAGERY

Richard Carolan

Dedicated to the adolescent addicts and the fire in their souls.

Introduction

The development of a mature "identity" involves the development of a consistent, coherent means of being in relationship with the world. It serves as a means of communing between the outer world and the inner world. Success in this process may often involve a great cost to the experience of the inner world. The "identity" only represents a portion of the human capacity. When internal voices that are not heard cry out in suffering, this is psychopathology. One area where there has been a historical "pathological" response to the process of human development is in the development of addiction.

Addiction and Identity

Addiction is recognized as a serious blight in our time, impacting social, cultural psychological, spiritual, and physical human development. The National Survey on Drug Abuse conducted in 2003 (United States Department of Health and Human Services, Substance Abuse and Mental Health Services Administration, n.d.a) identified that 9.1 percent of the total population age 12 or older were classified with substance dependence. This use and abuse of drugs occurs across the spectrum of the population; lifetime nonmedical use of pain relievers among persons over 12 is around 30,000,000 individuals. Alcohol is the most commonly used drug: 120,000,000 (over 50%) of the population aged 12 or older were current drinkers of alcohol, 54,000,000 were binge drinkers, 16,100,000 were heavy drinkers, and 47.8 percent of adults between the ages of 21 and 25 were binge drinkers. Over 30,000,000 drove under the influence of alcohol in 2003. In addition, those who abuse drugs are more likely to suffer from a severe mental illness. The 2003 survey showed that adults who used illicit drugs were more than twice as likely to have a serious mental illness and 20.6 percent of the youth between 12 and 17 received treatment for emotional problems in the year prior to the 2003 interviews.

While the prevalence and impact of substance abuse is startling, it is not a new phenomenon. The use of mind-altering substances has been a consistent part of the history of human development. Fifty thousand years ago, Neanderthals used medicinal and hallucinogenic plants. Alcohol is the most popular psychoactive drug throughout history; in fact, the earliest human crops were wheat and barley, grown for bread and beer. Wine was so prized in some Middle Eastern areas that important individuals were sometimes buried with their personal drinking cups. Many ancient cultures consider alcohol, particularly wine, a "gift from the gods." Yet as each culture developed, it went through periods of placing religious, social, and/or legal controls on the use of alcohol and other drugs. Inaba & Cohen (2004) describe the reasons that people throughout history have chosen to alter their perception of reality through the use of substances as the desire to:

• Ease fear and anxiety
• Reduce pain
• Treat illness
• Give pleasure
• Facilitate talking to gods
• Develop altered states of consciousness

There has been a marked increase in published research concerning addiction over the last few decades. While even as late as the early 1970s there was little published research on addiction. Currently, there are many publications that are updated on a daily basis (such as the internet publication of the Boston University School of Public Health, available at http://jointogether.org). Most of the research is on etiology, prevalence, and treatment. The incongruence between the persistent human drive towards mind-altering substances and the vast individual and community costs of abuse of these substances is seldom addressed (Truan, 1993). Some who argue that addiction is a disease might explain this incongruence; however, this is not a clear solution (Satel, 1999). The search for mind-altering experiences is part of the history of human evolution and part of the process of human development. It is critical to consider how the drive towards mind-altering experiences is intrinsic to the human experience and how this drive toward mind-altering experiences affects the developmental process of individuals.

Erikson's Stages

Erikson (1959/1980) identifies four stages of development that normally occur during the years when individuals are most active in the abuse of mind-altering substances, from the age of twelve years up through and including old age. Each of these stages involves the process of encountering tasks that have to do with developing and maintaining a clear and successful sense of self. The development of a clear identity is seen as an indicator of a healthy, evolving individual, whereas confusion in the developing of a clear, consistent identity is seen as a sign of pathology. There is tremendous pressure on the developing individual to identify and adhere to a clear sense of self. Deviations from this identity are seen as indicators of immaturity or pathology.

Erikson's fourth stage involves the encounter between identity vs. role confusion. This most often occurs between the ages of 12 and 18. During this period, every adolescent must examine his or her identity and the roles he or she must assume. The adolescent must develop an integrated sense of self (Bee & Boyd, 2003). There is a tremendous pressure during this time to develop a clear linear focus. While adolescence is one of the most creative periods of development, as demonstrated by the range and diversity of expressiveness in this period, the pressure for linear identity development tends to repress the imaginal in psychological development. While a certain degree of expressiveness is tolerated, there is the expectation and pressure towards a linear cohesion of a preferred identity. It is noteworthy that while most individuals have at least a degree of success in developing this "identity" during adolescence, 20.6 percent of the youth between 12 and 17 received treatment for emotional problems in the year prior to 2003 interviews (United States

Department of Health and Human Services, Substance Abuse and
Mental Health Services Administration, n.d.a). It is also noteworthy that
47.8 percent of adults between the age of 21 and 25 were binge drinkers,
and these individuals fall in the middle-age bracket of the next stage of
Erikson's developmental tasks, intimacy vs. isolation, occurring
between the ages of 18 and 30.

It is only after you have formed a clear identity that you can develop
intimacy and a kind of fusion with another. The individual in the
process of addiction is likely not progressing in the same manner along
these developmental tasks as one who is not in the process of addiction.
The addicted individual likely has a developing sober identity as well as
a developing intoxicated identity and perhaps an identity that mediates
between the two. The addict is often able to develop "successful" identities related to each of these renditions of the self, yet never fully
embraces either, tending toward isolation as opposed to intimacy.

In considering the theories of addiction as related to the process of
human development, it is of particular interest to look at the emphasis
in both the psychological and the spiritual models of treatment (Center
for Substance Abuse Treatment, 1999). These two models seem directly to address the issue of identity formation. The psychological model
suggests that addictive behaviors are attempts at destruction of the self
as a result of vulnerabilities in the ego. The spiritual model directly
emphasizes the limitations of the self and the need to go "beyond" the
self as a means of working with addiction. These theories of treatment
are interesting when contrasted with the tasks of human development
that postulate the need to develop a coherent, consistent sense of self.
The later two tasks and stages in Erikson's theory, generativity vs. stag-
nation (age 30 to old age) and integrity vs. despair (old age), also require
the development of the cohesive self for successful completion. Generativity is seen as reaching beyond the cohesive self towards others.
Integrity vs. despair is an interesting task because we are expected to
integrate the earlier stages of development to lead to integrity; however, if this integration leads to despair, then it is seen as pathology.

The question of what happens to the imaginal process (so alive in the
young child) as children grow older and pass through this stage of
development of identity is seldom addressed in the literature. The
process of human psychological development begins with fantasy and
play in the imaginal realm. According to Freud, the internal world is a
world of images, not thoughts (Levine, 1992). Jung sees the imaginative

process as the basic form of psychological process (Levine, 1992). As the child grows into adulthood, however, there is a tremendous pressure to leave behind the imaginal and to strive towards a rational, cohesive, linear self. While most individuals are successful at this process and develop an "identity," there is also a tremendous amount of suffering in the process, so much so that, as mentioned previously, in the early stages of "identity" development more than 20 percent of the individuals suffer from emotional problems and almost 50 percent are binge drinkers. It is clear that even while individuals develop this rational "identity" they are also driven toward experiences outside of that "identity." According to Hall (Hall & Nordby, 1973, p. 49);

> The person may become civilized, but he does so at the expense of decreasing the motive power for spontaneity, creativity, strong emotions, and deep insights. He cuts himself off from the wisdom of his instinctual nature, a wisdom that may be more profound than any learning or culture can provide. This can lead to the crisis of identity formation, and psychopathology.

Psychopathology is the study of the suffering of the psyche. Were we to recognize addiction as a psychopathology, then we would be responsible for studying the suffering of the addictive process. Nakken (1988) states "addiction is a direct assault against the self" (p. 54). He goes on to state, "addiction moves a person away from their self." While the moral model (Center for Substance Abuse Treatment, 1999) suggests that addiction is due to deficits in the characters of those who abuse substances, perhaps individuals use substances sometimes consciously and perhaps most often unconsciously due to deficits in the imaginal realm.

Maslow and the "Self"

Maslow (1968), in his chapter entitled "The Need to Know and the Fear of Knowing," identifies Freud's greatest discovery as the recognition that the cause of much psychological illness is the fear of knowledge of oneself (p. 60). He recognizes that in the process of developing "self," we end up with a dialectical relationship between fear and courage (Maslow, 1968, p. 67). It is interesting that Maslow describes acute identity experiences as "peak experiences"(p. 103). Maslow identifies characteristics of "peak experiences" and states that in his opinion, individuals while in "peak experience are *most* their identities" (p. 103). He then goes on to list some of the characteristics of "peak experiences":

. . . feels himself to be at the peak of his powers
. . . effortlessness and ease of functioning
. . . free of blocks inhibitions, cautions, fears
. . . more spontaneous, more expressive
. . . more uncontrolled and freely flowing outward
. . . most free of the past and the future

He goes on to say (p. 111) that "it *may* turn out that *only* "peakers" can achieve full identity" (his emphasis).

It is interesting to note that the above-mentioned characteristics are similar to what those using mind-altering substances describe as their experience while under the influence of the drugs. It might be suggested that those who abuse substances are seeking "peak experiences" beyond what they have attached to or seem to be within the capacity of their developed "identities."

This may be related to the distinction that Jung identified between the "self" and the "ego"; Jung sees the self as the center of the total personality. The ego, on the other hand, Jung regards as "the center of my field of consciousness" (Jung, 1970, p. 460).

According to Jacoby (1985), the self is "the invisible, central, ordering factor of the human psyche" (p. 197). He also refers to the self as the uniting of opposites. "Psychologically it might be said that the self gives the ego an assignment, a task to be performed" (p. 201).

The conflict may be between the "self" and the "ego" or between the "identity" and a multiplicity of internal experiences and imaginings that are not held in the capacity of the "identity." The result is pathology, a suffering of the psyche. This may also be a factor in substance use, abuse, and subsequent addiction. Mind-altering substances allow the capacity for imaginal experiences that are outside of the realm of the preferred "identity."

Identity, Treatment of Addiction, and the Imaginal Process

It is interesting to consider this in relationship to the history of addiction treatment in the United States. Currently, there is much emphasis on the dual-diagnosis model in the treatment of addiction. This development stems from the recognition that the suffering of those with substance abuse issues is highly correlated with those individuals who have other sufferings of the psyche. Historically, the Alcoholic Anonymous (A.A.) model of treatment has been prevalent in the U.S. This model has links to Jung as well as to concepts of the "self." Jung treated a client named Rowland H. for alcoholism and after failed treatment attempts, Jung supposedly told Rowland that his only hope was for a "spiritual awakening." Rowland took this message to a colleague named Ebby, who was also suffering from addiction, and Ebby took the message to his colleague, Bill Wilson. Bill Wilson was one of the founders of A.A. The message was that alcoholism created a spiritual void and what was required was a spiritual rebirth.

This, of course, led to the development of the "Twelve Steps." The first three steps of the twelve steps serve as their foundation. This is where most of the initial work is and it is often considered the most difficult work. The first three steps are:

Step 1. We admitted we were powerless over alcohol; that our lives had become unmanageable.

Step 2. Came to believe that a power greater than ourselves could restore us to sanity.

Step 3. Made a decision to turn our will and our lives over to the care of God as we understood Him.

These steps are interesting in light of the earlier discussion. This treatment approach is stating that our "identity" is not working, and in fact is not based on sanity. In order to establish sanity, we must let go of our "identity" and trust in something other than our "identity."

The twelve-step tradition identified this "something other" as "God as we understood Him." Another means of identifying this "something other" might be to recognize it as the imaginal capacity inherent in every human being. According to Levine (1992), emotional disorders are sufferings in the imaginary capacity and the cure can only come from a "renovation of the imagination itself" (p. 2). One might postulate that the drive that seems to be inherent in the human process of development towards the use of mind-altering substances might have its core in the drive to be in relationship with the imaginary capacity. Levine goes on to state "the therapeutic ideal would be a freeing of the imagination, the possibility of a more creative life for the person" (p. 2).

Our understanding of the process of individuation should perhaps be considered from a cost/benefits perspective. The developmental process can propel us towards a focused enhancement of one aspect of being while repressing or derailing us in others. Who has not reflected upon what happens to the wonder and "magic" in the imaginal world

of the healthy child as she moves into "maturity." We offer a momentary sigh for the "lost child," then move to appreciating her maturity
and developed "sense of self." While certainly a developed sense of self
is necessary to function in the adult world, does this developmental
process require the repression or derailment of imaginal capacity?
What happens to the undeveloped imaginal capacity? Might there be
relationship between this phenomenon and the over 20 percent occur-
rence of emotional disturbance in adolescents and the practice of binge
absorption of mind-altering substances in 50 percent of young adults?
Might there be a relationship also to the almost 10 percent of individuals who involve themselves in ingesting mind-altering substances even
to the degree that they reach a stage of powerlessness, and according to
the twelve-step approach, must surrender this developed sense of self to
another imagined capacity?

Thus far, we have only discussed and offered statistics related to the
addiction to mind-altering substances. There is also a long list of
pathologies related to addiction to mind-altering behaviors. There is
gambling addiction, sex addiction, eating addiction, Internet addiction,
and so on. It is likely that a considerable percentage of the population
is involved in mind-altering addictive behaviors as a means of engaging
in a way of being that allows an experience that is other than the experience of that carefully developed "sense of self." It seems that instead
of pathologizing the innate drive towards engagement in the imaginal
capacity, we should tend to it through a means that allows us to integrate it with the healthy sense of self.

The Arts and the Developmental Process

The human practice that is perhaps most rooted in the imagination is
the practice of making art (Levine, 1992). Freud and Jung have both
shown that the role of psychotherapy involves the healing of the imagination through the imagination (in Levine, 1992).

The arts can serve as an invaluable practice in facilitating the individual's engagement in his or her imaginal capacities. Through practice in
using the arts with a therapeutic focus, the developmental process of
developing "identity" can continue without the costs related to the
repression of imaginal capacities.

Art can also be used as a means of therapeutic intervention with
those individuals for whom the process of developing "identity" may

have had a cost that involves addictive patterns of behavior. A brief overview of art therapy and treatment orientations in substance abuse can highlight some of the potential in this area. Waller and Mahony (1999) discuss four primary areas where they see art therapy as playing a critical role in addiction treatment. These areas are:

• expression and communication of emotion
• loss of control
• low self-esteem
• isolation

Each of these areas can be seen as related to identity development and conflict related to the cost involved with coherence to a singular sense of self. Facilitating expression becomes an important issue because the developing individual who is abusing mind-altering substances often has a lack of awareness of thoughts and feelings. Conflicting emotions may be related to repression of the imaginal capacities, and issues related to this conflict are more accessible through image. The art process may also allow the individual to engage the imaginal being without activating the defenses of the ego. Art therapy can provide containment and safety for expression of repressed and/or difficult material. Distancing allowed through the art therapy process can lead to therapeutic imaginative process that does not threaten the developing "identity." The issue of "loss of control" when facilitated through the art process can be used as a means of growth instead of destructive experiences and suffering. Art, then, can serve as a means to emphasize and develop strengths through increasing capacity to experience emotions and engage with the imaginal capacity. Through the structured practices of art therapy, this can be done without threatening the development of "identity" and while increasing self-esteem.

The individual suffering with substance abuse has increased experience of isolation as the addiction develops. Through habitual use, the individual isolates from his or her positive development of "identity," and is also isolated from expanded use of imaginal capacities as he or she isolates from others. This isolation may, to some degree, be the result of attempts to engage the imaginal capacity, even while struggling to develop a healthy "identity." Art can serve as a means of facilitating the synergy of the imaginal self-developing in congruence with the development of "identity." Art can serve as a process of communication and social interaction that includes interactions in the imaginal realm. Universality of experience can be achieved through the art and art can serve to counteract emotional and psychological withdrawal from the developing self as well as from others.

Reviewing the above material reveals that art can be used in a therapeutic manner to engage the imaginal process in the development of "identity." The use of therapeutic art practice in a proactive manner may lessen the human drive towards mind-altering substances that serve as a means of quieting the hunger of repressed imaginal capacity.

Historically in the United States, the treatment of addiction has been primarily focused on the twelve steps. The twelve steps, as mentioned earlier in this chapter, originated from the theory that what was required to overcome addiction was a "spiritual awakening." The twelve-step process focuses on letting go of the "identity" through recognition of its powerlessness in dealing with addiction. What is required in the twelve steps is turning over one's will and one's life to "God as we understood him." Turning over one's "identity" to a higher power requires engagement in imaginal practices. Art can be used effectively as an imaginal practice that facilitates working with the twelve steps. There are numerous reports of strategies for using art therapy as a means of facilitating twelve-step work (Carrol, 1990; Julliard, 1999; Liao, 2002). These references primarily focus on specific interventions that are targeted toward the tasks of each of the twelve steps, the primary focus being on the first three steps. Additional consideration should be given to developing the practice of engagement with art in a therapeutic manner that facilitates activation and practice of working with the imagination. As discussed earlier, the art process could be a means of facilitating the individual's engagement in the imaginal capacities, which might be aligned to the "higher power" discussed by the twelve-step tradition. Through active engagement in the imaginal process, individuals might be able to develop practices that would counteract some of the costs involved in the process of developing a coherent "identity."

It is not at all clear that the imaginal process needs to be repressed in order to develop a coherent "identity." Perhaps the engagement with imaginal capacities could play a critical role in the development of "identity" while limiting the costs of this process. The development of the imaginal capacities concurrently with the development of "identity" might lessen the human drive towards mind-altering substances that facilitate the individual experiencing an alternate sense of self in the process of human development.

Example: Jesse.* Jesse is a 16-year-old Caucasian male in a residential treatment center for addiction. He has a dual diagnosis of marijuana dependence and depression. He had been in this treatment center for over six months. Jesse had little consistent childhood support in establishing his early childhood identity. One area where Jesse did feel that he was able to develop some sense of identity was through graffiti. Graffiti served Jesse as a means of being able to project an identity in the world, and to have a sense of control over that projection. He could develop a "tag" that would in some way be based in both his current identity and his fantasy about himself.

It was important to Jesse that he could use a means of expression and communication with which he felt comfortable and successful to serve as the methodology of self-exploration. For him, then, this was not a process of repression of the imaginal but a process of discovery through the imaginal.

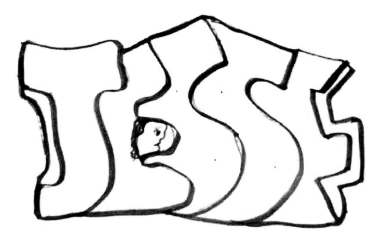

Figure 7.1. *Identity,* by Jesse.

In a later session, Jesse was asked to draw his past, present, and future. This directive fits well into the motivational enhancement approach (Center for Substance Abuse Treatment, 1999) to treating addiction, as it allows many opportunities for identifying and exploring ambivalence. Jesse worked on this theme over a couple of sessions and through the art was able to begin integrating experiences and possibil-

* Special thanks to Sarah Moffett for her work during her Notre Dame de Namur University internship experience and for relaying the case of Jesse to the author of this chapter.

ities. While there was little consistent support in his early childhood experiences, like many adolescents who do not have a lot of positive childhood memories to hold on to, Jesse is very protective of the memories he does have. His initial image of the past is a home that is most striking in how it reflects a self-portrait with large tears falling from the eyes/windows.

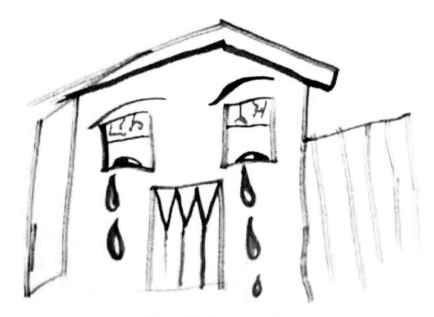

Figure 7.2. *Memories,* by Jesse.

Jesse was later able to use art as a means of transforming this old identity through some of what he currently experienced as strengths (his graffiti and his peer identity, which he associated with his "posse") and to imagine a future where these qualities were combined with his interest in working with kids through arts and crafts.

Working with his art therapist, Jesse was able to bridge his comfort with graffiti images into a process of using art materials to reflect on himself and his life. He was developing awareness of his thoughts and feelings and reversing the repression of imaginal capacities. The art therapy process was allowing containment and safety for the expression of difficult material without activating the defenses of the ego.

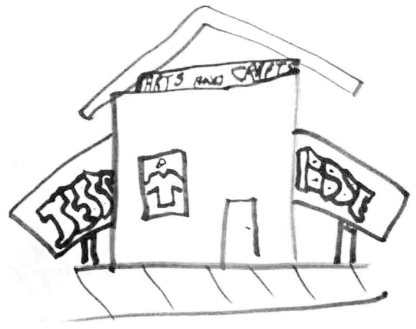

Figure 7.3. *All Together,* by Jesse.

In a later session, the art therapist facilitated Jesse in the process of developing a "me-box." This simple directive is very powerful in allowing a multiplicity of images of the self to be held in one presentation. The process and the product acknowledge that there are multiple aspects and images of the self, some of which are part of the "identity" that is established in the world and some of which are not. In his "me-box," Jesse included a carcass of a deer being fought over by two animals. He described this as his two sides battling over his future and whether or not he would use and engage in addiction and criminal acts. This image depicts the conflict between the "sober identity," the "using identity," and the young person trapped between the two. It reveals the intensity and confusion of drives and conflicts that were jumbled within Jesse at this time when there was so much pressure on him to commit to an acceptable identity.

Jesse's work continues in the treatment program, as it will continue when he leaves. He has, while in treatment, learned new means of developing his imaginal capacities while simultaneously developing a strength-based identity. Through the use of art therapy, adolescents are

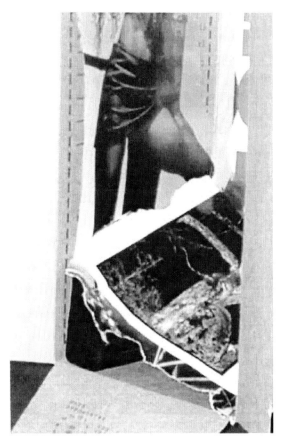

Figure 7.4. *My Me Box,* by Jesse.

able to engage alternative ways of knowing and facing the "crisis" of their development. Jesse, like many other adolescents in addiction treatment, often depicts the addiction as an overpowering monster.

The art therapist worked with Jesse through art and creativity in empowering him to imagine other possibilities in his relationship with this "monster." Once the "monster" was externalized through art/imagery, the possibilities of understanding and engaging with this "identity" were enhanced and could be stimulating and empowering. Jesse was able to take advantage of this process through identifying and working with another of his images, which at first he identified as a predator; he was later able to transform this "identity" from a predator to an ally. This "identity" now serves him in getting his needs met and developing a more accurate vision of future possibilities.

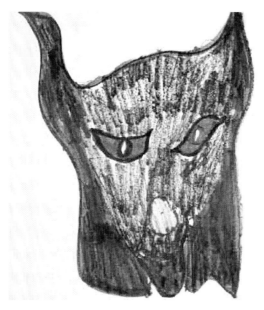

Figure 7.5. *The Monster Within,* by Jesse.

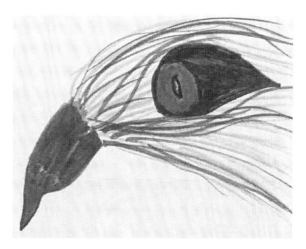

Figure 7.6. *A Helper,* by Jesse.

Jesse has, through art, begun the process of developing a relationship with the "monster" within himself, in the hope of not repressing but channeling its forces in the work of developing his identity. He has a great deal of work left to do in working with his addiction as well as in continuing with the development of his identity. Through the use of the art process, with the guidance of an art therapist, Jesse has begun to access his imaginal capacities in a manner that can serve him and empower him in venturing with more confidence and openness into the possibilities of experiencing and identity development.

The field of addiction treatment is beginning to make some progress in recognizing the therapeutic powers of the creative art therapies. The program that Jesse is attending has an art therapist as a consultant as well as art therapy interns working with the male and female adolescents in both individual and group therapy. The program also has an ongoing mural program that helps the clients to take ownership of the program and the images that inform the therapeutic community. The creative art therapy component of the program also involves trapeze arts, poetry writing/readings, and a digital self-story creation program. The treatment program also has a strong wilderness component in which art therapy plays a significant role. Art therapy can play an important role in countering the imaginative repression that too often becomes linked with the development of a coherent identity, as well as offering creative, growth-oriented alternatives to the use of mind-altering substances as a means of allowing alternative identities to find and maintain a voice of expression.

Bibliography

Bee, H., & Boyd, D. (2003). *Lifespan development* (3rd ed.). Boston: Allyn and Bacon.

Carrol, C.A. (1990). *Use of the twelve steps of Alcoholics Anonymous in art therapy with substance abusers.* Unpublished master's thesis, College of Notre Dame (currently Notre Dame de Namur University), Belmont, CA.

Center for Substance Abuse Treatment. (1999). *Enhancing motivation for change in substance abuse treatment.* Treatment Improvement Protocol (TIP) Series, Number 35, DHHS Pub. No. (SMA) 05-4081. Rockville, MD: Substance Abuse and Mental Health Services Administration.

Cushman, P. (1990). Why the self is empty: Toward a historically situated psychology. *American Psychologist, 45,* 599–611.

Erikson, E. H. (1980). *Identity and the life cycle.* New York: W. W. Norton. (Original work published 1959.)

Erikson, E. (1963). *Childhood and society* (2nd ed). New York: W. W. Norton.

Hall, C. S., & Nordby, V. J. A. (1973). *Primer of Jungian psychology.* New York: Mentor.

Inaba, D. S., & Cohen, W. (2004). *Uppers, downers, all arounders: Physical and mental effects of psychoactive drugs* (5th ed.). Ashland, OR: CNS Publications.

Jacoby, M. A. (1985). *Longing for paradise.* Boston: Sigo.

Julliard, K. (1999) *The twelve steps and art therapy.* Mundelein, IL: American Art Therapy Association.

Jung, C. G. (1970). *Collected works* (Vol. 6). Princeton NJ: Princeton University Press.

Lasch, C. (1978) *The culture of narcissism: American life in an age of diminishing expectations.* New York: W. W. Norton.

Levine, S. (1992). *Poiesis: The language of psychology and the speech of the soul.* London: Jessica Kingsley Publishers.

Liao, P. L. (2002). *Art therapy for the first three steps of AA's 12-step program.* Unpublished master's thesis, Notre Dame de Namur University, Belmont, CA.

Marcia, J. E. (1980). Identity in adolescence. In J. Adelson (Ed.), *Handbook of adolescent psychology* (pp. 159–187). New York: Wiley.

Maslow, A. (1968). *Toward a psychology of being* (2nd ed.). New York: Van Nostrand Reinhold.

Merriam-Webster Online. (n.d.). Retrieved from http://www.m-w.com/dictionary/identity

Nakken, C., N. (1988). *The addictive personality: Understanding compulsion in our lives.* New York: Harper Collins.

United States Department of Health and Human Services, Substance Abuse and Mental Health Services Administration. (n.d.a). *National survey on drug use and health* (NSDUH)–*Homepage.* (n.d.b.) Retrieved from https://nsduhweb.rti.org

United States Department of Health and Human Services, Substance Abuse and Mental Health Services Administration. (n.d.b). *National survey on drug use and health.* Retrieved from http://www.oas.samhsa.gov/nsduh.htm

Satel, S. (1999, Winter). The fallacies of no-fault addiction. *Public Interest, 134*(99), 52.

Truan, F. (1993). Addiction as a social construction: A post empirical view. *Journal of Psychology, 127*(5), 494.

Waller, D., & Mahony, J. (1999). *Treatment of addiction.* London and New York: Routledge.

Westin, D., & Heim, A. K. (2005). Disturbances of self and identity in personality disorders. In M. Leary and J. P. Tangney (Eds.), *Handbook of self and identity* (pp. 643–664). New York: Guilford.

White, W. (1998). *Slaying the dragon: The history of addiction treatment and recovery in America.* Bloomington, IL: A Chestnut Health System Publication.

Chapter 8

THE SPARKS OF ADOLESCENCE

Arnell Etherington

Dedicated to Billy Etherington, whose life inspired me.

The Story Begins

Alice[1] was 15 when her troubles came to the attention of the author-ities. At this middle stage of adolescence she was facing develop-mental issues similar to those faced by other 15-year-olds. Her questions included "Who am I?" and "Where do I fit in?"

Alice had recently transformed into a young woman bearing all the marks of adolescent sexuality and verve. She dressed in black with short skirts, tall boots, low-cut blouses, and red-black lipstick. She was outspoken and aggressive, yet depressed. Her parents, both of whom she knew, had never married. Her father lived several thousand miles away. His life involved a series of partners. Her mother lived, unhappi-ly, as a single woman, with the patient's great-grandmother. At the time of her treatment, Alice lived in her mother's household with three gen-erations of women.

Life for Alice began insecurely with her mother. After Alice was about 6 years of age, her father visited her only infrequently. As she developed and began to have problems at school and at home, she faced her first traumatic experience. She was perfunctorily shipped off to her father as a kind of unspoken punishment. It was as if her mother had run out of options and needed a break from parenting. Rejected by

---

1. Alice is a composite case illustrated with art by the author.

mother, Alice would live with her father for about a year, have problems, and then parental rejection would be repeated and she would be sent back to her mother's house.

This sequence resulted in Alice's attachment and schooling being interrupted by moves back and forth between her parents' homes over the next 9 years. Alice was her parents' pawn. However, she appeared to care for both parents until they set limits or insisted on house rules, then they would become the focus of her contempt.

Adolescent Physical, Social, and Psychological Growth

Adolescence begins with a review of the previous phase, latency. The latency-age child, despite involvement in school and with friends, is emotionally still firmly rooted in the family. The cornerstone of good parenting is for both parents to provide a secure base from which the adolescent can make exits out into the world and return, knowing for sure that he or she will be welcomed upon return, nourished physically and emotionally, comforted if distressed, and reassured if frightened (Bowlby, cited in Lanyado & Horne, 1999). In early adolescence this pattern is disrupted by the normal distancing from parents and the corresponding turning to the peer group (Weideman, 1975). As the adolescent gets older, she ventures farther and farther from home base for longer periods of time. The more the adolescent can count on that base, the more confident she is (Lanyado & Horne, 1999). Alice was already in the middle stage of her adolescent development and her early years had been fraught with unexpected and traumatic transitions in her home base.

Adolescent Physical Growth

Adolescence (itself) begins with biology and ends with psychology. It is kick started by puberty, cruising slowly to a halt at adult identity; the point at which the petrol is getting low and there is a need to think about saving some for the long, straight road ahead. (Van Heeswyk, cited in Lanyado & Horne, 1999, p. 38)

Shifts in the body self in pre-puberty will often be marked by regression back to the safety of previous experience when the individual is facing the adolescent tasks (Lanyado & Horne, 1999).

Intimacy adaptations and action around the body come to the fore in adolescence. Unfortunately, due to the haphazard course each unique adolescent takes through these years, there is no comparability between specific ages. For example, the 9-year-old who begins to menstruate is quite different from the 16-year-old who hopes that any day her period will commence. The boy whose growth spurt comes much later than that of his peers may find the idea of coping as an adult to be terrifying and bizarre. Although adolescence is often seen as a tumultuous period, most young people make their way through fairly successfully, despite projections of adult envy and adult fears with each step (Lanyado & Horne, 1999).

Somehow, adapting emotionally means making parental intimacies less intense—a reworking of the Oedipal experience. Intimacy of mind and body are at play, as the adolescent can be perceived as beginning to take over from the parent responsibility for and ownership of his or her body at a time when the earliest sexual feelings of infancy are revived (Lanyado & Horne, 1999). Indeed, ". . . puberty is a biological event with profound psychological repercussions" (Weideman, 1975, p. 189).

Today, through the general availability of books, movies, and the Internet, adolescents may be exposed to sexual information and experiences often far beyond their physical experience or even their personal desires. They come to their first experiences with some ideals of how things should work and may be devastated if their experiences do not "fit the picture." Adolescents begin to address their sexuality with masturbation in the privacy of their own worlds and move quickly into the intimacy of masturbating with a partner. Social pressure and lack of social control can lead to early intercourse. Most adolescents want any experience that their peers are having, yet they fiercely want the event to be personally fulfilling, or at least experienced on their own terms. The move toward choosing and selecting sexual partners and then considering marriage can be a long and circuitous road.

Simultaneously with moving toward more intimate and physical relationships, in adolescence there also begins a separation from parental ideas and opinions. The parent may feel suddenly in the cold as the adolescent, a separate entity, begins his or her path towards being more alone and separate in the world.

Early Adolescent Phase

In the early adolescent phase there may be a reluctance to care for the body, whereas in later adolescence great attention and concern for the body may commence. Experimenting with drugs, alcohol, nicotine, sports, and sex are all ways of interacting with the body. These items and events can pull the adolescent back to early mechanisms for dealing with the unmanageable and also give time to rehearse for possible futures. The ability to tolerate this new, fluid body self is crucial (Lanyado & Horne, 1999). It is not surprising that this is a time when eating disorders and suicide occur among those who find the move toward an adult sexual self too difficult, if not impossible.

The movement into peer groups and developing independent relationships with adults other than their parents takes on greater weight in early and mid-adolescence than at earlier ages. The adolescent at this age may develop a "crush" on the opposite or same-sex adult or peer.

Socialization with a group in middle adolescence is similar in function to the relationship with a close, same-sex friend in early adolescence. "The mirroring obtained from peers is important at this stage and is based on the early identity formation of infant years" (Lanyado & Horne, 1999, p. 39). The group, in its diversity, offers a variety of roles as models and shared experiences of responsibility and irresponsibility. The peer context takes on primary value to the adolescent trying out different aspects of the self and perceiving them in other members of the peer group. Thus, risk-taking can be indulged and has the flavor of the omnipotence of the toddler age, a heady disregard for anything dangerous with the belief that it will never strike personally. Failure in friendships and relationships at this developmental stage becomes a handicap for attempting to try patterns out in the world. These types of failures often impede further development.

Middle Adolescent Phase

Developmentally, middle adolescence is when heavier educational burdens are placed on the young. Intellectual challenges become serious and the adolescent sees achievement or failure in very black-and-white terms. The effects of these successes or failures are incorporated into the adolescent's emerging identity (Jessor, 1993). As with many aspects of adolescent development, trouble in one arena can dangerously polarize the whole sense of self. The adolescent can become quite rigid in his or her all-or-nothing thinking, making it hard to keep the younger child part of the adolescent alive, the part in which transitioning phases can be so creative.

Late Adolescent Phase

Theoretically, the securely attached late adolescent will acquire a stable identity. Most clinicians consider that adulthood is firmly planted in an individual by about 25 years of age. No longer conflicted by the parental relationships, the young person can find a more disengaged intimacy with the family, allowing for the ease of coming and going as well as family appreciation. With securely attached children, this can occur from a position of security as a separate, functioning young adult (Lanyado & Horne, 1999).

Identity

The need for an identity is stronger in adolescence than in any other time of the life cycle. As the adolescent faces external, physiological, and internal pressures concerning the future, the subtext of all that occurs is, "What will I be?" (Lanyado & Horne, 1999). The adolescent's task is to establish, through trying on a variety of roles, an adult identity. Erikson (1959) has given us ample insight into the social developmental stage of identity versus identity confusion. When we don't know who we are, our behaviors will be a surprise. The therapist, for example, often experiences in clinical work the surprise of an adolescent who may find him- or herself on probation and wondering, how did this happen? Identity, as an adult, is core to self-hood, but without it we flounder and depend on others to set us straight on whom we are and where are we going. Near the end of adolescence, there is the beginning of a settling on that identity.

Adolescent Intellectual Growth

The adolescent years include the potential for an expansion of the intellectual capacity for abstract thinking. Piaget's (1954) theory of the cognitive stages of development emphasizes that at adolescence the young person will, over an eight- to ten-year period, move from a concrete to a formal stage of thought. The concrete stage is characterized by thought in terms of categories and graded series. In early adolescence, a shift begins where thought forms of ordered matrixes of all the possibilities inherent in the system begin to be used. "One sees a shift from thought about 'things' to a vastly expanded capacity for thought about words, concepts, thoughts, hypotheses, ideas" (Weideman, 1975,

p. 198). In childhood, problem solving is organized almost exclusively around concrete actualities. In the formal stage of abstract thinking, the full range of possibilities comes to the fore. Thus, there is a full breadth of thinking about things that might be or might develop but are not yet the case. The delinquent or insecurely attached adolescent is often one whose capacity for abstraction is undeveloped, since he or she has become stuck or overinvested in direct concrete action (Weideman, 1975). The thinking transition of this developmental level often comes directly into play when parents and children argue. For example, the adolescent who says she has "cleaned her room" has concretely gone in and moved around certain pieces of clothing or dishes or bed sheets. The parent, however, has held a whole range of ideas in his or her abstract concept of "clean your room."

Adolescent Spiritual Growth

Spirituality is a common facet of adolescent lives. In adolescence, that part of self begins to blossom, and holds a sense of wonder, influencing both their choice of peer groups and behavior (Holder et al., 2000). Often the young adolescent will find a spiritual or religious teen group to be a relief from the academically competitive peer group at school. In a spiritual group, there is often a mix of ages and the emphasis is on peace, harmony, conflict resolution, global issues, caring for one another, as well as doing good deeds. This type of group not only instills in the adolescent the ideals of an inner faith but also serves as a platform for ethical and moral discussion that may never arise in other peer groups. The adolescent, asking questions about the meaning of life and death, finds that this transitional group from family to society offers a time and a place for exploring these rich topics. Adolescence is also a time when one can be put in the vulnerable position of being pulled to a group that, while also social, may be harmful, such as a cult or gang. These groupings often insist on maintaining a parental type of control over the teen's life with the lure of group dynamics and a philosophy that initially sounds like something the adolescent wants.

Adolescent Creative Growth

The adolescent, with a changing identity, risk-taking propensity, and interest in exploring greater parts of him- or herself, is likely to fall into creative work as long as there is freedom in the context. In creative expression, the individual adolescent finds that the schemas used for themes in latency are less interesting or even too restrictive. The artwork of an adolescent has the potential for becoming more passionate and expressive. Their appreciation of the work is different. Creative expression allows for and fosters fantasy. Expressive fantasy becomes an aid in facing the difficult tasks of adolescence. There is often a resurgence of expression during this period.

> As Blos (1962) points out, teenage diaries and journals are good examples of this process. The healthy youngster is able to find ways of explaining and experimenting with identity concerns by harnessing the creativity that will help his/her transition from child to adult. (Linesch, 1988, p. 6)

The adolescent is capable of more self-directed work than usual home and school routines allow. Adolescents are ready to learn more skill. "Art is regarded personally and developmentally, as a mode of assimilating and giving form to experience that is significant to the artist" (Lindstrom, 1957, p. 85). Art serves well for therapeutic expression because the adolescent enjoys it. Art expression is a developmentally appropriate modality that provides adolescents with an ego-syntonic aid in their difficult struggles (Linesch, 1988).

The Story Continues

Alice, having lived through early parental rejection, was facing developmental changes in her physical, psychological, social, intellectual, and spiritual selves. Making this transition on her own was more than she could handle. Alice came to the day treatment center after an incident of fire-setting in which she intentionally burned down the shack next to her home.

The profile for the adolescent fire-setter is a serious one. Though the ratio of fire-setters is 6 to 1, male to female, for both it can be a path to more serious behaviors. "Often the female fire-setter will do it for excitement and amusement" (Perrin-Wallqvist & Norlander, 2003, p. 151). A retrospective study of the charts of 13 female adolescent fire-setters revealed severe family and individual pathology (Sanders & Awad, 1991). In reviewing Alice's case, her fire-setting was a cry for help that could be heard outside of her family. Without intervention, it was likely to be repeated.

The etiology of moderate fire-setting often involves conduct problems such as disobedience and aggressiveness. It may be accompanied by an experience of anger and resentment over parental rejection. Adolescent fire-setters who move into residential care are more likely to come from single-parent homes, display increased delinquent behaviors, "show greater depressive symptoms, and report more aggressive thoughts than outpatient adolescents" (Pollinger, Samuels, & Stadolnik, 2005, p. 345). Recidivism has been associated with little discipline, family conflicts, limited parental acceptance, and/or neglectful family environment. It may be that the patient has experienced a crisis that reduces stress tolerance and that the increase in impulsivity leaves him or her vulnerable to such activities as fire-setting (Slavkin & Fineman, 2000). Certainly Alice had faced these issues in her history. With Alice, it was understood that family therapy had to be part of her treatment. She was a bright young woman who was at grade level, so she began treatment in the day treatment program, which consisted of therapy and school on an isolated campus. Verbal therapy, activity therapy, or group art therapy took place 5 days a week. The program included weekly individual therapy, weekly family therapy, and crisis intervention whenever needed. Directives relating to family, self, problems, and imagination were included in the art therapy group and individual treatment plans. Clients were encouraged to use art materials, paints, pencils, collage, and clay for these ideas. Examples of the directives follow:

- With your parent's separation, what problems did you face?
- What problems did you face as a child in a family that was separated?
- How does it make you feel that your parents do not live together?
- What part of your life do you spend with your father?
- What part of your life do you spend with your mother??
- Can you represent your ideal relationship with your mother?
- Can you represent your ideal relationship with your father?
- Can you represent your ideal relationship with grandparents? And your extended family on both sides?
- Looking at your physical, psychological, social, intellectual, and spiritual well-being, how does it feel to be in trouble and how does it feel to be out of trouble?
- What is it like to be your age?
- If you were to select a helper animal, what kind would that be and what would the qualities be that would be helpful to you?

- Can you draw why?
- Find an image that represents your success in life (in the program, in your therapy).
- Make a mask, using an animal that represents some part of you.

Alice's adjustment to treatment was slow. She was appropriately cautious. Why should she trust any adults? Those closest to her had rejected her again and again. Rejection is a difficult experience when you are not sure who you are and you are wanting so badly to stand on your own two feet and yell "I am."

It was established at the beginning of her treatment that Alice had no experience of physical or sexual abuse. She was, however, asked, "What problems do you face?" Figure 8.1 represents her answer: "I'm pissed cuz no one will let me say anything." The gag may represent a profound sense of being silenced against her will or just of never being heard. The piece, done in black, possibly reflecting her depression, represents a girl with no hands to grasp what she wants and needs in the world, who is gagged and frowning about the situation. The sadness is that Alice wishes to speak, yet in her mind there is no one willing to listen.

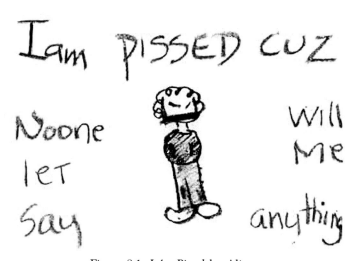

Figure 8.1. *I Am Pissed,* by Alice.

Up to this point the staff had been unclear that Alice had anything to say. She was often quiet and withdrawn. This piece and her willingness to represent it became the opening to articulate her voice, her will, her wants and her needs, as well as her frustration and anger, particularly with her family and school.

Children and adolescents who set fires are angry. The act of setting fires precludes the verbal expression of the fire-setter's thoughts and feelings. But certainly it is a way that identifies the individual as finding only pathological and/or primitive means to express his or her personhood.

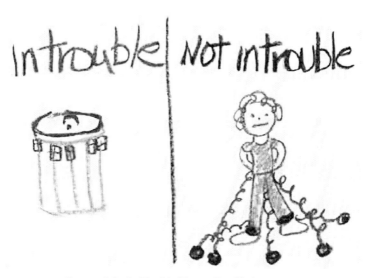

Figure 8.2. *In Trouble/Not in Trouble,* by Alice.

In Figure 8.2, Alice answers the question, "How do you feel when you are in trouble and when you are out of trouble?" Neither image looks at all comfortable. "Not in Trouble" appears as worrisome and as restricted as "In Trouble." The image of the locked-down garbage can versus the ball-and-chained girl immediately gives one a sense of unfair restriction or of needing enormous external control in order to maintain appropriate behaviors in the world. The image may raise the question of whether she feels she needs this control on some level. Or, is it an image of what she believes others think of her or what others in authority positions do to her? These questions remain unanswered, but the piece certainly appears to be a protest.

Alice's mother began to work in family therapy and was committed to seeing Alice through her crisis. She contracted not to send Alice back to her father should Alice regress and agreed that visits with her father would be regularly scheduled regardless of Alice's behavior. Several months later, Alice engaged in a collage about her "helper animal." She was asked to choose an animal that could be a helper to her and to express in words and pictures the qualities this animal held for her. Alice chose a dolphin and called her collage "Dolphins of Life" (see Figure 8. 3). Her dolphins engaged in a number of activities. One picture on the collage illustrates a dolphin and the trainer feeding the dolphin. The dolphin may be jumping to the trainer's command. It is a picture of nurturance, yet the obedience is unclear. Middle adolescents probably understand less than the dolphin does about what they need to do to make a relationship with individuals in authority work on their behalf. Here might be the consummate image of coming home to receive the nurturing and feeding one desires. A second picture shows the human with his underwater gear down under the water building a relationship with the dolphin in the dolphin's environment. The human actually adapts to go into the dolphin's space, to meet the dolphins as they are in their environment. Here the human is confined and the dolphin is free. This may be part of Alice's wish for a parent to enter into her life and be with her on her terms. Or, it may show her wish for the parent to feel the restrictions she has felt as Alice wanders free.

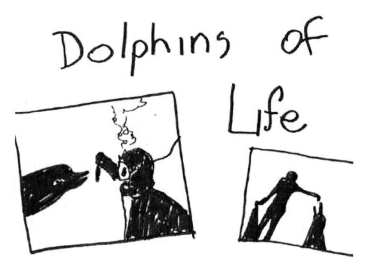

Figure 8.3. *Dolphins of Life*, by Alice.

In another photo (not shown), two dolphins find partnership with just one other dolphin in the sea. This may reflect Alice's continuing search and gesture to find reliable and predictable trust with one or the other of her parents. She may hope for that return to an earlier developmental phase when one is close to one's parent all the time, or even together in a symbiotic relationship.

Over the next year, the image of the dolphin seemed to speak to Alice because again and again she used the image in some way to tell her story. In Figure 8.4, several dolphins are pictured jumping together in synchronized form in the open sea. Alice had been asked to find an image for her ideal relationship. These dolphins may reflect a family or her peer group working together. Here the dolphins are free (momentarily) of their watery home and flying through the air. They do this activity naturally in the wild, and Alice may be coming closer to seeing that relationships do not have to be pushed in order to be effective, fun, loving, and truthful.

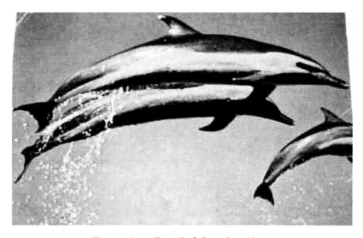

Figure 8.4. *Four Dolphins,* by Alice.

Another image (not shown) shows four dolphins being touched by a crowd as they jump out of the water. This image was placed inside a Self Box, reflecting parts of Alice's inner self. She chose this image at a time when she was at the height of her arguments with her mother regarding home rules and consequences. Alice and her mother had moved their arguments into the therapy hour, which gave them the confinement and help they needed to come to a resolution. The dolphins in this image are contained in a pool at an amusement arena where they live. This speaks again of the two challenges an adolescent faces: adjustment to the collective and finding a comfortable place in the collective where one can be oneself. Here the dolphins live in a confined and artificial environment and are not free to roam as they wish. The confinement that the family places upon each adolescent may be experienced as comfortable and safe at one moment and as oppressive and controlling the next. For the adult in the adult world, however, this is a dichotomy that most adults manage.

Later in the Story

About 18 months into treatment, Alice chose the image of a dolphin jumping through a flaming hoop in a free collage. The photo was central to the piece, and may represent what is at the center of things for Alice.

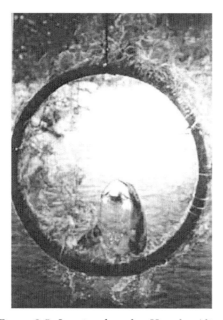

Figure 8.5. *Jumping through a Hoop,* by Alice.

For a fire-setting patient, this is a poignant picture. The animal here has learned to attend to the flames and the heat but not to be burned by the fire. In a sense, the dolphin conquers the fire. The fire here is contained and the animal can jump through it without its destructive impulses taking over. The animal must use its intellect and senses as well as control its body to execute this move. So too can adolescents use these aspects of themselves to achieve their goals. In fact, the audience, similar to the collective watching an adolescent successfully achieve developmental steps, probably applauds the dolphin as it jumps. However, in this photo the attention is only on the dolphin as it performs its task at hand, which may reflect Alice's focus on the intellectual and emotional work to which she has been attending.

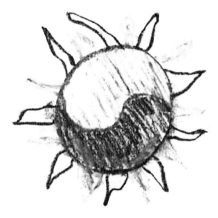

Figure 8.6. *Dark and Light,* by Alice.

Near the end of therapeutic day treatment, Alice was asked in art therapy to make a symbol representing her success in the program. She made a yin/yang symbol with flames around the outside (Figure 8.6). The yin/yang symbolizes balance of the male and female energy in the universe. For Alice, it represented a "soothing image where dark and light go together." She made no comment about the surrounding flames. Perhaps now her internal flames could be calmed in this image of balance. Alice was now ready to begin reintegration back in a high school off campus. She had no further incidents of fire-setting. Her depression and aggression were both reduced. Her mother became a more effective and committed parent. Her great-grandmother became less intrusive in her mother's life. Alice visited her father on a predictable, scheduled timetable. She began to have deep friendships with her peers and showed responsible behaviors.

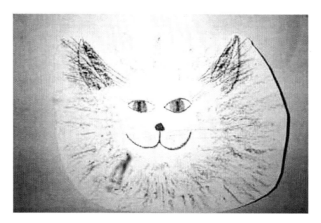

Figure 8.7. *A Happy Kitten,* by Alice.

Alice's final image before leaving day treatment was a mask drawing of a kitten (Figure 8.7). The kitten looks happy and a little mischievous. The kitten is a soft and feminine image that up to this point might have been too vulnerable for Alice to reflect. It is an animal that likes to curl up and be petted on its own terms and yet is rather independent of its owner. Hopefully, Alice is beginning to feel more comfortable living in her day-to-day existence as she enters the later phases of adolescence.

The Story Moves On

Joseph Campbell in *Myths to Live By* (1972) speaks about the fact that humans, of all the animals, have one of the longest gestation periods to adulthood. "For the human infant is born–biologically considered– some ten to twelve years too soon. . . . The young . . . born too soon . . . have the home which is again a sort of external second womb" (pp. 44–45). The home "womb" must be a reliable and consistent place in which to experience the developmental phases leading to adulthood. Adolescence is the last step before adulthood and for that reason is of vital importance. When a home "womb" is dysfunctional or unavailable, community resources must step in.

When dealing with children and adolescents who have experienced some parental separation or the trauma of parental neglect, abuse, or abandonment, safety and protective factors found in therapeutic right-hemisphere feeling experiences are essential to restructuring their brains and behavior. Art therapists and neuroscientists are now identifying art as a vehicle for treating trauma and connecting feelings with thoughts. For Alice, working in art with a knowledgeable helper in a safe and protected environment allowed her to look at her life story, forgive her family and herself, and make sense of her life journey—so far.

References

Blos, P. (1962). *On adolescents, a psychoanalytic interpretation*. New York: Free Press of Glencoe.

Campbell, J. (1972). *Myths to live by*. New York: The Viking Press, Inc.

Erikson, E. (1959). *Identity and the life cycle*. New York: International Universities Press.

Holder, D. W., DuRant, R. H., Harris, T. L., Daniel, J. H., Obeidallah, D., & Goodman, E. (2000). The association between spirituality and voluntary sexual activity. *Journal of Adolescent Health, 16*(4), 295–302.

Jessor, R. (1993). Successful adolescent development among youth in high-risk settings. *American Psychologist, 48,* 117–126.

Lanyado, M., & Horne, A. (Eds.). (1999). *The handbook of child and adolescent psychotherapy*. New York: Rutledge.

Lindstrom, M. (1957). *Children's art*. Berkeley, CA: University of California Press.

Linesch, D. (1988). *Adolescent art therapy*. New York: Brunner/Mazel.

Perrin-Wallqvist, R., & Norlander, T. (2003). Fire setting and playing with fire during childhood and adolescence: Interview studies of 18-year-old male draftees and 18–19-year-old female pupils. *Legal and Criminological Psychology, 8,* 151–157.

Piaget, J. (1954). *The construction of reality in the child*. New York: Basic Books.

Pollinger, J, Samuels, L., & Stadolnik, R. (2005, Summer). A comparative study of the behavioral, personality, fire history characteristics of residential and outpatient adolescents (ages 12–17) with fire setting behaviors. *Adolescence, 40,* 345–353.

Sanders, E. B, & Awad, G. A. (1991). Adolescent female fire setters. *Canada Journal of Psychiatry, 36*(6), 401–404.

Slavkin, M., & Fineman, K. (2000, Winter). What every professional who works with adolescents should know about fire setters. *Adolescence, 35,* 759–774.

Weideman, G. (1975). *Personality development and deviation*. New York: International Universities Press.

Chapter 9

THE DEVIANT ADOLESCENT: CREATING HEALTHY INTERACTIONS AND RELABELING THROUGH ART THERAPY

David Gussak

Dedicated to my daughter, Samantha Rose, who is coming into those interesting transitional years of adolescence.

Introduction

The trend toward teen violence and delinquency is one of the most vexing and enduring faced in contemporary society. The pervasiveness of the problems delinquency creates has been answered through the institutionalization of increasingly large numbers of disaffected teenagers. Understanding how adolescents experience institutional life is a matter of importance to their care, and to society. Those who work with institutionalized adolescents have much to learn about how they influence the behavior of teenagers in their care. Society has not quite grasped how adolescents who are labeled delinquents or deviants continue to maintain these identities through their interactions in society. While negative interactions can perpetuate these behaviors, certain positive interactions may help reverse these tendencies. This chapter will summarize the interactionist perspective and its relationship to the study of deviance and delinquency. It will then discuss the institutionalization of the disaffected youth, present self-appraisal and labeling theories within this context, and ultimately use these theories to explore and explain how the act of creating art and art therapy can be used to help reverse this trend. Vignettes will illustrate this viewpoint.

The theories of interactionism emerged from the philosophies of James, Cooley, Dewey, Mead, and Blumer. At the beginning of the twentieth century, psychology pioneer William James claimed that the social self is developed through the interaction of the individual and social groups (James, 1890/1918). Cooley (1964) saw ". . . interactionism as a framework through which social reality was to be interpreted" (p. 9) and believed that a joint interdependence between the social environment and individuals exists. People interpret what others see in them by noting the actions with those with whom they interact; ". . . the self emerges in a process of communication and interaction as the individual responds to and internalizes aspects of ways others have of acting toward the person" (Hall, 1981, p. 50). Dewey (1930) maintained that people, their environments, and their thoughts are interconnected to form a larger whole.

As early as 1964, Mead argued that the self develops through its interactions and activities within social experiences. It is the interactions of the self that actually define situations. The self develops from the ". . . process of social experience and activity . . . [that] develops in the given individual as a result of his relations to that process as a whole and to other individuals within that process" (p. 199). The self not only interacts with others, but also with one's own thoughts and ideas through self-reflection. This notion that the self is created and defined through interactions with no corporeal objects is similar to Blumer's (1969) theoretical perspective of interactionism.

Blumer (1969) claimed that in an interaction, a person will interpret other people's gestures and will then act on what he or she perceives the meaning to be from this translation. Stressing the importance of the interaction between both people and objects, he continues, noting that objects have meaning for people. Meaning is ". . . not intrinsic to the object but arises from how the person is initially prepared to act toward it" (Blumer, 1969, pp. 68–69). Objects, on the other hand, include ideas and thoughts as well as things that are tangible. It is the sharing of these objects, and the interpretations thereof, that define the action and interaction between people. Those who subscribe to interactionism claim that meaning emerges from the interaction between people (and objects). Thus, meanings and interpretations are social products. Ideas lead to action and the construction of a practice and/or product.

It is through these interpretations that a societal context and the roles of the people that make up this society–including teenagers–are defined. Simply put, interactions define people. Therefore, meanings and interpretations are social products. Such actions are also maintained through self-appraisals and societal categorical definitions, or what we define as labeling.

Self-appraisal and Labeling

Role taking is an important aspect of interactionism (Blumer, 1969). This consists of "projecting oneself into the role of others, and appraising from their standpoint the situation, oneself in the situation, and possible lines of action" (Bartusch & Matsueda, 1996, p. 147). This influences how one views oneself and can ultimately sway one's self-concept and identity. Once this identity is acted upon, and if negative behavior ensues, the labeling that occurs perpetuates this identity, creating a cycle that is difficult to break (Becker, 1963/1991). What has been discovered, however, is that labeling a child as delinquent or simply "bad" may be more of a result of the child's economic background, and may include those who are socially-economically disadvantaged or of a minority group (Bartusch & Matsueda, 1996). It is not clear if such labeling influences the self-image more if it is a "formal" label (i.e., derived through the courts, schools, or psychiatric or detention facilities) or an informal label (i.e., given by peers and family). Paternoster and Iovanni (1989) stress that it is more important to focus on informal rather than official descriptors. One thing is clear: regardless of the type of label, labeling influences self-appraisals, and in turn, perpetuates delinquent and deviant tendencies.

Deviance and Delinquency

Rules and sanctions against those that violate the rules, and thus the norms, are created through social acts, note Lauer and Handel (1977). Many people cooperate and contribute to sanctions. Deviants, or those that belong to a deviant group, are those who have been sanctioned. "Normal" or normative groups define social problems. "Social norms are two-sided. A prescription implies the existence of a prohibition and vice-versa. . . . Norms that define legitimate practices also implicitly define illegitimate practices" (Cloward & Ohlin, 2001, p. 359). By simply creating a standard of acceptance, society is indicating that anyone that engages in behavior out of the boundaries of this prescribed standard is deviant.

Social problems, according to Spector and Kitsuse (1973), emerge through assertions of grievances and claims from members of a group or a society. "Behaviors are not recognized as deviant, or criminal, unless others, as members of cultural groups, react to them as such" (Hagan, 2001, p. 6). Merton explained deviance through what he labeled the "strain theory"; simply clarified, if people are unable to meet their goals through acceptable means, they may try to achieve these goals through deviant means. For example, when individuals or groups discover that "no matter how hard they work or try, they cannot achieve the levels of satisfaction or material wealth to which they have been taught to aspire, deviant behaviour may be the result" (Merton, cited in Rouncefield, 2003, p. 8).

Definitions of deviance, however, are not clear-cut, and many theoretical perspectives exist (Becker, 1963/1991). What the definitions and perspectives all seem to have in common is their belief that any member or part of society that tends to reduce stability is considered deviant. Ultimately, deviants belong to the groups within our society that do not fit in. Deviants are the "outsiders."

Much like Spector and Kitsuse, Becker believed that society was responsible for creating, or defining, deviance. Sagarin (1975), for example, notes that deviance is attributed to people, and behaviors, that provoke hostile reactions. He makes a distinction between deviance and criminality, indicating that on occasion deviance and crime overlap. Therefore, there are some people and behaviors that are both criminal and deviant, others that are deviant but not criminal, and still others that are criminal but not deviant. For the sake of this chapter, the development of deviance will correspond with that of delinquent or offending tendencies.

Granted, as Hagan (2001) pointed out, the problem with relying on labeling theory to explain the genesis of deviant behavior is that it puts the entire responsibility for such anomies on society and disregards biological and psychological impulses. As Hagan notes, we can assume that a more proper explanation of the causation of deviance and delinquent tendencies is a combination of the two—the natural impulse may have been present, but societal interactions perpetuated and maintained the deviant tendencies. Dryfoos (1996) outlined six significant risk factors that have been deemed factors for initiating and perpetuating deviant behaviors. They are: (a) poor parenting, (b) interactions in school and response to the schooling process, (c) peer influences, (d) psychological difficulties such as depression or bipolar tendencies, (e) living in an impoverished and crime-ridden neighborhood, and (f) ethnic behaviors and discrimination, i.e., neighborhood gang participation. Four of the six risk factors involve societal and environmental interactions and all factors influence interaction and labeling to instigate and perpetuate deviant tendencies.

Deviant adolescents act out and express their anger and frustration in dangerous and unacceptable ways–that is, unacceptable by society's standards. This, in turn, can cause retribution or punishment and sanctions by societal members, including the institutionalization of these disaffected youths in detention facilities. Such invalidation of these feelings may cause the adolescent to form further self-perceptions as a deviant, perpetuating a cycle.

According to the interactionist perspective, deviant behaviors may be learned through observation and through interaction with other deviants, either within institutions or on the streets. This is similar to the process by which gang members operate, or the phenomenon that happens in juvenile and adult correctional facilities where newer inhabitants learn continual deviant behavior, in some cases necessary for survival, from those who are more institutionalized. It is the "normative behavioral systems of groups that support, encourage, and condone violence" (Vigil, 2003). Such behaviors are not only accepted within that subculture but are expected. Such interactions also create an identity within the adolescent, one that is difficult to replace with one that is more acceptable to the larger society.

Thus, simply "locking someone up" may not only be insufficient, but may very well continue the cycle through strengthening the deviant self-appraisal, as Rubington and Weinberg (2002) indicated. The deviant identity is maintained through an interactive process between those that break the rules and those that enforce them. The punishment does not deter the behavior but does in fact confirm for the perpetrators that indeed, they are deviant; "how others respond is therefore crucial to the process of acquiring a deviant identity" (Brownfield & Thompson, 2005, p. 23).

Reinforcing or Reversing Labels: The Interaction of Art Therapy

As social interaction creates, defines, and maintains deviant behavior, so it can also help remove the deviant label and interrupt the cycle of unacceptable behavior. It is through interaction that new behaviors and identities can be developed and validated, thus redefining, reversing, or halting the actions of those considered deviant or delinquent. According to Gussak (in press), "The art therapist uses the art-making process to aid in developing appropriate interactions and decrease aggressive tendencies."

Symbolic interaction can occur between people and objects as well as between two people, notes Blumer (1969). He continues, ". . . objects– all objects–are social products in that they are formed and transformed by the defining process that takes place in social interaction" (pp. 68–69). Actions and interactions are initiated and reinforced through the active interpretation of noncorporeal objects. What is more, societal norms can be defined through the shared meanings of objects, connections, and interactions.

Through visual cues, art is used to create and define interactive relationships. For example, art is a prevalent form of communication and definition between members of adolescent street gangs. These gang members communicate through several different visual cues including hand gestures, color codes, and graffiti (Jackson & McBride, 1986). Graffiti images are used to create an identity, a sense of belonging, and a means of communication within the gang. They are designed to separate the gang set from rival gangs or outsiders (Huff, 1990; Padilla, 1992). Different gangs have different lettering styles and the images become stylized and intricate, taking on the form of self-labeling within the gang. "Taggers" (graffiti artists) are well-respected within their own groups. To "strike out" a gang sign or gang member's logo is considered a high insult. A challenge to the turf is grounds for serious retaliation. Gang members are even willing to die to protect the integrity of their own visual identity (Decker & van Winkle, 1996).

Images demand respect. Honoring the visual cues, in essence, values the members. By using images to communicate and connect group members, positive interactions become more likely. Padilla (1992) indicated that some gang members want to become legitimate, accepted into our society, but they have been embroiled in a subculture for so long they may not know how to separate themselves for acceptance into the conventional society.

Experience with gang members and "gang wannabes" in a therapeutic context proves complicated. (Gang wannabes, wanting to be gang members, take on gang attributes but are not yet gang members–some believe that wannabes are more dangerous than actual gang members, as they may have more to prove). They choose to interact primarily with those in their own group because, according to gang members, those outside their group clearly do not understand or accept them. Occasionally, when time, personnel, and right-hemisphere materials such as art, music, sports, and writing are provided, new forms of communication develop, new ways of self-expression emerge, and the individual is able to discover a sense of his or her real self.

Therapists, coaches, and community leaders in their authoritative communities can and should incorporate into their interactions with deviant children and adolescents these natural tendencies for acceptance, connection, and identity. This is a natural growth out of art therapy. Introducing art materials for creative expression to clients considered delinquent creates a new interaction, and a new social pattern. Interacting with the materials and the art product, clients will begin to redefine their images, and eventually will be acceptable to others. Where previously the deviant individual had difficulty connecting with others, when he or she is using the art materials, the individual's previous label becomes blurred. It is at this time that a new sense of self is created, occurring through the client's connection to the art, the therapist, and the process. Specifically, the deviant person may now be identified as "an artist" as well. The client and the therapist now belong in the same socially acceptable context, the art world, constructed and maintained through the shared conventions of the collective media. A new relationship is established between the artist and the therapist (Becker, 1982). Teaching a client how to use art materials for self-expression creates a new mode of interaction. Mastery of the materials promotes a new sense of self-worth apart from previously established hostile and deviant identity.

Case Studies[1]

RICK.[2] Rick was an 11-year-old boy who was in a behavioral health facility for "acting out" and aggressive tendencies. He was proud that he belonged to a gang. His deviant behavior was initiated and maintained

---

1. All names have been changed.
2. Rick was previously introduced in *Art Therapy and Social Action* (in press), in the chapter entitled "Alleviating Aggression through Art Therapy: A Social Interactionism Perspective."

through continual support for these behaviors from his gang peers, and through the strong reaction and sanctioned labels provided by the staff at the facility. He was seen as a deviant and delinquent. He did little to convince the facility otherwise. It was not until new labels were created for Rick that he was able eventually to construct a new identity. Through art, Rick was able to create a new label, with a more appropriate and healthy self-appraisal.

Rick constantly "tagged" his gang moniker on the walls of the unit in which he was housed. As there was a rule against displaying gang insignias, let alone writing on the walls, he frequently got in trouble with the facility's staff. He became angry when the graffiti was washed off the walls, and several times, he attacked those who were cleaning up the drawings. Rick perceived touching his art as an act of disrespect, and as evidence that staff did not accept who he was.

After several other similar interactions, after receiving permission from the unit administrator, I made a deal with Rick. I first reminded him of the hospital regulations and then told him that if he agreed to work with me, he could do the gang tags on separate paper and keep them in his desk drawer. He also had to promise that he would not hang the drawings up. He agreed to this, and he spent several afternoons drawing quietly with pencils on white paper. Each drawing was meticulously completed. After he completed several of these drawings, I then suggested that instead of illustrating his gang's name, he do a drawing of the name his gang called him. Eventually, the drawing evolved into an embellishment of his real name. These he showed proudly, and they were hung on the wall in his room. By the time he left the unit, he was much more compliant with staff directives and was decidedly less aggressive than before. Through this process, Rick was validated. He formed a self-label that was deemed "acceptable." Concurrently, his behavior was altered to conform to social norms and his own concept of himself was strengthened. He developed a healthier self-appraisal, and saw himself as an individual within a different societal context.

The art therapy process provides a means to interrupt the cycles of deviance and delinquency by strengthening a sense of self, providing an avenue to express negative emotions in an acceptable and appropriate manner, creating new meanings, and tapping into empathic responses (Gussak, 1997, 2004; Gussak, Chapman, Van Duinan, & Rosal, 2003). While it is common to believe that the client creates an art piece with little thought to the viewer, all artists take into account what the viewer may think of the result: "It is crucial that, by and large, people act with the anticipated reactions of others in mind. This implies that artists create their work, at least in part, by anticipating how other people will respond, emotionally and cognitively, to what they do" (Becker, 1982, p. 200).

KEVIN:[3] When the artist creates an image with hostile content, he or she may be doing it as a means to "attack" the viewer. Art, however, is an acceptable way to express hostility and the therapist can use the pictures to promote acceptance and success. As sessions continue, the client understands that these images, and by extension the client, are accepted. Once a client feels validated, the images may begin to evolve into more complex and thought-inducing products. For example, Kevin was a 17-year-old biracial resident of a juvenile detention facility (his mother was white and his father was African-American). Kevin had sporadic contact with his father, who was addicted to drugs; he saw his mother often, but she was considered "nice but a pushover" by her son. His biracial parents were responsible for one of Kevin's initial difficulties. For example, he was often made fun of by the peers on his unit for his lack of racial identity. He constantly talked about being confused with his own sense of self: "I feel like I don't belong." In a sense, he seemed to be missing a label.

Kevin's initial arrest was for drug-related activities, i.e., possession, consumption, and distribution. His drug history on the street was quite extensive. Even in the facility, Kevin used illicit drugs, or found unique methods to take his medication inappropriately, such as "snorting his aspirin." Recognized by the staff of the facility as being difficult, he was subsequently labeled a deviant. For his part, Kevin seemed to reinforce this label through displaying inappropriate attention-seeking behavior. For example, he told his peers on the unit that his sister had been kidnapped. He also told them that his family lived in New Orleans and was unreachable after Katrina, the hurricane that affected the region in the autumn of 2005. When staff and peers voiced sympathy and pity, he laughed, letting them know that he was only kidding. He seemed to be trying to develop a new label.

---

3. Special thanks to Jody Teixeira for her work during her Florida State University internship experience and for relaying the case of Kevin to the author for this chapter.

If he thought he was being wronged or disrespected, Kevin became angry. Generally, his anger just resulted in him grinding his teeth and clenching his jaw. If his anger persisted, it developed into "acting out" behavior, most commonly through verbal abuse and threats. Several times his angry outbursts and threats resulted in days added to his sentence.

Kevin enjoyed doing art and working with the art therapists at the facility, when he had an opportunity to articulate his personal issues, but initially he drew gang symbols that were inappropriate and against the facility rules. When asked to write or draw advertisements about who he was or to focus on his self-identity, he often had difficulties. He was unable to complete the art and became frustrated, demonstrating the difficulty of not having a clear label for himself. Nevertheless, it was the art experience that made the difference. One art therapist worked patiently with him, helping him use media to express his feelings. Eventually, respect and a strong rapport were built between them.

After approximately 7 months in the facility, Kevin completed (Figure 9.1) a black-and-white painting of a large dragon attacking a tiny person; the stick-person is ineffectively shooting the dragon with a bow and arrow.

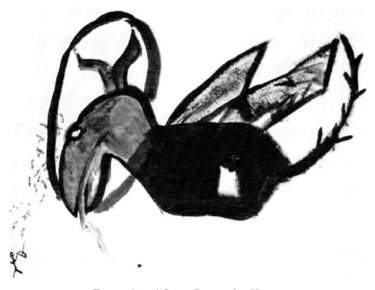

Figure 9.1. *A Large Dragon,* by Kevin.

After completing it, the drawing helped Kevin to understand that he was the dragon, specifically representing what he is like when he gets angry. He indicated, "When I get angry, it's like I grow horns." He pointed out to the art therapist what the individual components of the drawing represented–the white on the tips of the horn is hate, as is the white part of the stomach. The white part (hate) in his stomach comes out his mouth past his tongue, and gets vomited out, which he pointed out manifests into cursing and acting out. Yet, the art piece is hopeful–Kevin said the gray area in his head is new. It is where he is working on his anger, and the round shape around his head is the shield he puts up to protect him from the projectiles that the stick figure is shooting at him. Although he was somewhat unclear on whom the stick figure is, it is most likely "a peer who was kissing up with the staff." He did not provide additional information, but appeared satisfied with how the image expressed his feelings.

Kevin was able to process this piece with the art therapist, who accepted what Kevin said and consequently accepted him. This piece represented a turning point for Kevin, and he began to use the art process to express his feelings and to see his work validated by someone he valued. As a result, Kevin demonstrated an authentic representation of himself without fear of rejection.

Kevin, of course, did not demonstrate total understanding or give total information. At times, he still made inappropriate decisions. For example, after he discovered that he would soon be leaving the facility, he created a "hit list" of all the people he was going to kill, complete with dates and location. He did this as a means to extend his sentence. He told the art therapist that he was afraid to leave, as his parents did not effectively provide for him, and that he was reluctant to go back to the streets, back to his gang. The art therapist worked with Kevin in art to address these feelings and develop options rather than let Kevin extend his stay at the facility due to deviant behavior. In short, Kevin felt validated by the art therapist and by the art-making process. Subsequently, he was able to begin altering his own negative self-appraisal.

In Rick and Kevin's cases, the art process was used to initiate the reversal of negative labeling and poor self-appraisal. What became evident is that not only can the art process facilitate change in an individual; it can also facilitate change in a group label.

Changing a Group Label

Art therapy sessions were conducted in a special-needs, behaviorally focused school in a poor, rural section of the Florida panhandle. The school provided education to approximately 60 students, ranging in age from 12 to 18. The students, primarily African-American, were placed in this school after they had been removed from their previous schools for severely deviant behavior, including assault, drug violations, and larceny. Many of the students either belonged to street gangs or were gang wannabes. Often they were territorial and strongly aligned with their school districts, even when they denigrated the schools and the teachers from those districts. Although the students were placed in this school to avoid juvenile jail time, many of the students were still in the court system, awaiting sentences for various violations. Because these students were from different schools within this particular county, there were often conflicts based on territorial issues. Although teachers and behavioral specialists were taught conflict management, a security guard and often a county sheriff were assigned to the campus.

Because the majority of the students were seen throughout the school year in art therapy sessions unless they had been removed from the school to do some time in a juvenile correctional facility, or were deemed appropriate enough to return to the public school, the students saw the session as "just another class." Throughout the year, the art activities generally focused on individual tasks, addressing anger management, problem solving, and socialization skills. Rarely could the students work together to produce a group project. Some of the older students were able to construct simple group paper sculptures or take part in pass-around drawings, but these activities were infrequently attempted. It took a long time for rapport to be built within and between the students, and even then, it was a tentative rapprochement. However, ten weeks before the end of the school year, it was announced to the students that they would all participate in a mural that would be painted directly on the activities room wall. All of the students became excited about the idea of painting on a wall and they agreed to the established rules of the group. These rules focused on appropriate behavior, a decrease in aggression towards others in the group, following directions, respecting each other's space while painting, and respecting the materials. Of course, the most important rule was to respect the art therapist, and to listen to what he had to say. The students understood that if these rules were broken, the offender could not return to the mural. The students readily agreed.

With approximately 60 students, a system was established in which all of the students would plan, organize, and work on the mural in their respective groups rather than work together all at once. Although this approach had some drawbacks, including the real possibility that some things they were working on in one session might be altered prior to the next, it was believed that the drawbacks were far outweighed by the need for safety. They were all told of the possibility that something they worked on could be painted over and that the mural belonged to all the students at the school, and they all had the right to make changes. Again, surprisingly, they begrudgingly agreed to this, and proceeded.

The first step was to design the mural that would go on the selected walls. Each group of 6 to 10 students was provided butcher-block paper, and encouraged to draw a scene of their choice using oil pastels, colored pencils, and markers. In these drawings, the art therapists and faculty looked for consistencies and discussed with all of the group members what was emerging as the final theme. Surprisingly, without knowing what the other groups drew, all five groups drew a beach scene. There were differences. One had a palm tree. One had an overlarge sun with sunglasses (Figure 9.2), and one had a hut with a man fishing off a pier.

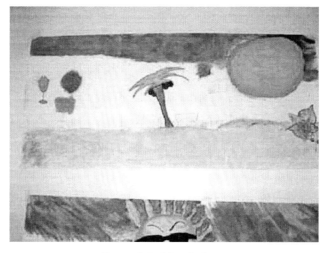

Figure 9.2. Mural ideas.

The similarities simplified the planning of the mural. During the course of the year, group members had recognized others in the group as being artistic. With the assistance of the art therapist, his intern,[4] and help from two of these students, the drawings were roughly outlined on the walls. The initial drawing was kept to a simple outline with few details to provide flexibility for the participants. For the next six weeks, all of the students painted the mural, making many changes, painting and repainting various details, ultimately covering the walls with a large extended beach scene (Figures 9.3–9.6).

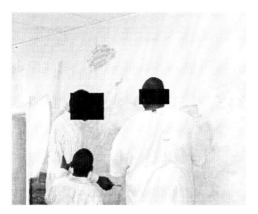

Figure 9.3. Students working on beach scene mural.

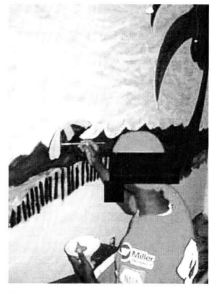

Figure 9.4. Students working on beach scene mural.

4. Special thanks to Florida State University student Kate Dorsey for her work as an art therapy intern during this project.

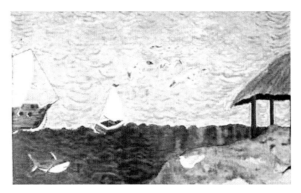

Figure 9.5. Beach scene mural.

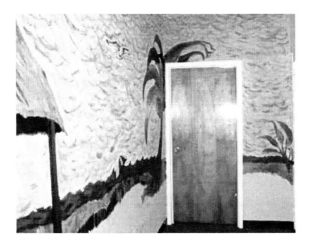

Figure 9.6. Beach scene mural.

Creating the mural was not without difficulties. Three of the participants were asked to leave the groups, and despite warning, there were
times when several of them became upset that what they had completed previously had been changed. There were days when much cajoling
by staff was needed to get them to focus on the task. Overall, redirection became the norm. Eventually these difficulties were eclipsed by the
successes.

Most of the participants, regardless of their territorial affiliations or
prior difficulties, were able to cooperate and work together. One student, who up until the creation of this mural had been obstinate, aggressive, and hostile, became a leader, offering to help some of the younger
students. He often would stick around and help the art therapists clean

up. When others became belligerent, he would talk with them to get them to calm down.

Many of the students claimed ownership, even when their contribution was as simple as painting the beige tones for the sand. This ownership was encouraged. At one point, one of the participants began painting his name and stylized lettering of his hometown, possibly evidence of gang relations. A peer, one that he was close to, told him to stop it, and brought his deviant behavior to the attention of the art therapist. With only a little resistance, the offender repainted the section. The offender also expressed pleasure when told that the names of all of the participants would be on the mural. At the mural's completion, the students proudly showed their work to the faculty and staff, who in turn greatly complimented their efforts and the finished product.

Overall, the mural activity proved successful in creating new interactions that provided some initial steps in reversing the individual labeling. Those who participated developed a sense of pride and identity as participants in an activity that was not only acceptable, but also encouraged, by the faculty and parents. The participants' self-appraisals were more positive, as evidenced by their pride in displaying their work and their eagerness to have their names included on the mural. Granted, this one project did not reverse what years of societal, familial, and institutional interactions had instilled, but it did provide a glimpse of the power that collaborative projects such as this might have helped to reverse labels of deviance, increase self-esteem, and provide a sense of acceptance within societal norms.

Conclusion

Through social interactions, people are labeled. Through these labels, the roles of social participants are defined, including adolescents who have been branded deviant or delinquent. Such labels, maintained through self-appraisals, make it difficult to break the cycle that may eventually be reinforced through institutionalization. The art therapist, with his or her unique skills, can facilitate new interactions; aid in relabeling people, and through validating can reinforce both new behaviors and identities. Art therapy can assist in reversing the labels associated with deviance and delinquency.

Art therapy itself is an "authoritative community" providing connections to materials, to others, and to self, all components necessary to the ultimate ending of the cycle of deviant identity. The therapist validates and reinforces new behaviors and identities. The art process assists in revising labels associated with deviance and delinquency and the art product establishes a positive self-appraisal. Through it all, the client learns to use art positively in personal and social communication and connections.

References

Bartusch, D. J., & Matsueda, R.L. (1996). Gender, reflected appraisals, and labeling: A cross-group test of an interactionist theory of delinquency. *Social Forces, 75*(1), 145–176.

Becker, H. S. (1982). *Art worlds*. Berkeley, CA: University of California Press.

Becker, H. S. (1991). *Outsiders: Studies in the sociology of deviance*. New York: The Free Press. (Original work published 1963)

Blumer, H. (1969). *Symbolic interactionism: Perspective and method*. Berkeley, CA: University of California Press.

Brownfield, D., & Thompson, K. (2005). Self-concept and delinquency: The effects of reflected appraisals by parents and peers. *Western Criminology Review, 6*(1), 22–29.

Cloward, R. A., & Ohlin, L. E. (2001). Illegitimate means and delinquent subcultures. In B. R. E. Wright & R. B. McNeal, Jr. (Eds.), *Boundaries: Readings in deviance, crime and criminal justice* (pp. 359–380). Boston: Pearson Custom .

Cooley, C. H. (1964). *Human nature and the social order*. New York: Schocken.

Decker, S. H., & Van Winkle, B. (1996). *Life in the gang: Family, friends, and violence*. Cambridge: Cambridge University.

Dewey, J. (1930). *Human nature and conduct: An introduction to social psychology:* New York: The Modern Library.

Dryfoos, J. G. (1996). Adolescents at risk: Shaping programs to fit the need. *The Journal of Negro Education, 65*(1), 5–18.

Gussak, D. (in press). Symbolic interactionism, aggression, and art therapy. In F. Kaplan (Ed.), *Art therapy and social action*. London: Jessica Kingsley.

Gussak, D. (1997). Breaking through barriers: Art therapy in prisons. In D. Gussak & E. Virshup (Eds.), *Drawing time: Art therapy in prisons and other correctional settings* (pp. 1–11). Chicago, IL: Magnolia Street Publishers.

Gussak, D. (2004). A pilot research study on the efficacy of art therapy with prison inmates. *The Arts in Psychotherapy, 31*(4), 245–259.

Gussak, D., Chapman, L., Van Duinan, T., & Rosal, M. (2003). *Plenary session: Witnessing aggression and violence-Responding creatively*. Paper presented at the annual conference of the American Art Therapy Association, Chicago.

Hagan, J. (2001). Seven approaches to the definition of crime and deviance. In B. R. E. Wright & R. B. McNeal, Jr. (Eds.), *Boundaries: Readings in deviance, crime and criminal justice* (pp. 1–12). Boston: Pearson Custom Publishing.

Hall, P. (1981). Structuring symbolic interaction: Communication and power. *Communication Yearbook, 4,* 49–60.

Huff, C. R. (Ed.). (1990). *Gangs in America*. Newbury, CA: Sage Publications, Inc.

Jackson, R. K., & McBride, W. D. (1986). *Understanding street gangs*. Placerville, CA: Custom Publishing Co.

James, W. (1918). *The principles of psychology* (Vols. 1–2). New York: Henry Holt and Company. (Original work published 1890)

Lauer, R. H., & Handel, W. H. (1977). *The theory and application of symbolic interactionism*. Boston: Houghton Mifflin.

Mead, G. H. (1964). *On social psychology*. Chicago: University of Chicago Press.

Padilla, F. M. (1992). *The gang as an American enterprise*. New Brunswick, NJ: Rutgers University Press.

Paternoster, R., & Iovanni, L. (1989). The labeling perspective and delinquency: An elaboration of the theory and assessment of the evidence. *Justice Quarterly, 6,* 359–394.

Rouncefield, P. (2003). *Robert Merton-Strain theory*. Retrieved January 26, 2006, from http://www.homestead.com/rouncefield/files/a_soc_dev_14.htm

Rubington, E., & Weinberg, M. (2002). *Deviance: The interactionist perspective*. Boston: Allyn and Bacon.

Sagarin, E. (1975). *Deviants and deviance: An introduction to the study of disvalued people and behavior*. New York: Praeger Publishers.

Spector, M., & Kitsuse, J. I. (1973). Social problems: A re-formulation. *Social Problems, 21*(3), 145–159.

Vigil, J. D. (2003). Urban violence and street gangs. *Annual Review of Anthropology, 32,* 225–242.

Chapter 10

FAMILY ART THERAPY:
REFLECTION, PROCESS, AND EVOLUTION

Anna Riley Hiscox

Dedicated to Shirley Riley, who through her words, deeds, and
visual way of knowing, taught me about art therapy.

Introduction

Belonging to a family is a universal facet of humanity. A family is
made up of people in "any intimate relationship, or parent-child
relationship, in which people live together, at least some of the time,
with personal commitments to each other, and who identify themselves
as an intimate group" (Shehan & Kammeyer, 1996, p. 425). Families are
generally open or closed systems. They generally do not seek counseling until they have reached an impasse where they believe that all the
solutions to their problems have been exhausted. When families no
longer have the elasticity to reach solutions through compromise, dysfunctional self-protective mechanisms begin to operate, separating family members into compartmentalized groups. The intolerable friction
between members is what is then presented in therapy as a family crisis. The premise of reshaping one's life within the realm of one's family is an exploratory process for the family and the art psychotherapist.
My approach is to integrate the theory and applications of the family
therapy pioneers with art therapy, creating what Riley (1994) calls an
integrated approach. This collaborative approach to working with families empowers families to use their strength to combat the self-destruc-
tive behaviors that have brought them to therapy. Understanding the

value of an integrative approach is the foundation for the development of a comprehensive treatment plan for healthier living.

In this chapter, the pioneering work of Mayer and Salovey (1990) on emotional intelligence and Goleman's (1995) book, *Emotional Intelligence,* will be discussed as they apply to art therapy theory and technique. Readers will observe how emotional intelligence can be abridged when violence, ineffective communication, and lack of empathy are the predominate characteristics of family functioning. Assessing family strength and resiliency through image will also be explored.

Family violence has kept pace with societal violence, impacting families of all races, nationalities, and social economic status. Therefore, creative avenues for healing in violent families will be discussed with the hope that continued research in the field of art therapy will diminish family violence and provide alternative avenues for healing.

I have worked with many families over the years that have been so overwhelmed with anger, secrets, and fear that their art expression was inexplicable. My goal is to assist families in repairing and reconstructing a family ego that is so damaged that a third eye (therapist) is needed to help stabilize and normalize family functioning. To these families, I say thank-you for showing me the way. I have also been blessed to live in a phenomenal part of the country where things are not always what they appear to be with respect to families. I was raised on the East Coast, where I was taught to believe that one's family of origin was "family." However, after adopting the West Coast as home, I have come to understand that "family" can be more than one's family of origin. My experience has helped me become open to the diversity of family formulation as defined by individuals who form family constellations.

Riley (1994) discusses the practice of co-construction, where therapist and client work together offering alternatives to the client for assuming a capacity to shape his or her own life (p. 5). This style of engaging clients allows family constellations to release, without guilt, the emotions they may harbor about members who no longer represent the family's values, ethics, and morals.

Over the years that I have helped families to reconstruct their lives, I have found that the major issues that are affecting families today have to do with feeling vulnerable within one's own family, the perception of (or lack of) respect, and physical and emotional abuse. When family members are unable to talk to each other, and are unable to show empathy, this lack of respect and abuse are then unconsciously transmitted intergenerationally. Therefore, communication is a major family issue to address in session, whether or not it is the presenting issue, because it is the voices of those involved that build a healthy or unhealthy family. Gottman's study of successful couples shows that "positive communication is based on old-fashioned good manners" more than anything else (cited in Wexler, 2004, p. 171).

Nonviolent Communication: Family Empowerment

Healthy families understand the concept of respect. They are active listeners and are able to give each other positive feedback and suggestions for optimizing family communication and interaction. In her book, *Nonviolent Communication,* Rosenberg (2003) postulates the theory of nonviolent communication (NVC) and states that when we are "replacing old patterns of defending, withdrawing, or attacking in the face of judgment and criticism, we come to perceive ourselves and others, as well as our intentions and relationships, in a new light" (p. 3). We "perceive relationships in a new light when we use NVC to hear our own deeper needs and those of others" (p. 3). Distressed families resort to counseling as a means of holding the family together when communication breaks down and family members are left with dysfunctional, abusive patterns based on emotional critiques and judgments. As Gottman (cited in Wexler, 2004) indicates, the major deficit in families with ineffective communication is lack of respect, i.e., respect for self and respect for others, which is a simple, old-fashioned manner. When respect is honored, individuals are able to be attentive and to show empathy. According to Rosenberg, the honoring of respect engenders a mutual desire to give from the heart.

Family Empowerment and Empathy

Empowering families with low frustration tolerance, deficits in problem solving, and difficulties with stated and unstated family rules requires a paradigm shift that involves the commitment of each family member combined with the creative astuteness of the art therapist. New family rules may have to be created and family members may have to grapple with letting go of the rules set forth by maternal and paternal relatives. For example, when parents command children to do chores and are met with resistance and questioned, "Why?", the parental retort, "Just because I said so," represents an archaic way of relating to children based on hierarchy, and should be replaced with reasonable explanations, intelligent rules, and expectations. In general, parents as heads of household are no longer required to live by family of origin rules. Conversely, art therapists should also keep in mind that cultural proclivities, although outmoded, may be important in maintaining family homeostasis. Assessing for and teaching empathic response is another major strategy that can be used to empower distressed families.

Families that function in a crisis mode may have members who have never developed empathy in childhood and, therefore, may not show compassion for others as adults. Consequently, the lack of empathetic response and compassion may be passed on to subsequent members of the family. The development of empathy depends on cognitive and language development, but it is also "supported by temperament and social experiences" (Berk, 1999, p. 373). Empathy is the ability to understand and relate to another person's feelings. A prerequisite for the development of empathy is the ability to feel and identify one's own feelings. Distressed families may be unable to impart this sensitivity. According to Hein (2005), sensitivity also means being receptive to others' cues, particularly nonverbal ones such as facial expressions. Hein posits that higher emotional sensitivity and awareness lead to higher levels of empathy. This leads to higher levels of understanding, which then leads to higher levels of compassion. Therefore, the family art psychotherapist has to wear many hats, including those of educator and collaborator in changing family dynamics. Working with families to develop emotional maturity can, in fact, rekindle underlying propensities toward violence and abuse. The therapist has to be skilled in anger management in order to reframe contentious thoughts to enable change in behavior, and to encourage empathy and compassion. The development of emotional intelligence is what is necessary for families in abject crisis.

To recapitulate, empathy is important to family systems and it underlies many facets of moral judgment and action. Many domestic violence theorists have surmised that empathy is a trait missing in abusive families. Goleman (1995) contends, "There is a psychological fault line common to rapists, child molesters, and perpetrators of family violence alike: they are incapable of empathy" (p. 106). The utter lack of empathy for the victims is one of the main focuses of new treatment being devised for child molesters and other such offenders. This chapter will also highlight the path one teenager is taking to heal from abuse and the lack of empathy in her family.

Emotional Intelligence

In 1990, Peter Salovey, along with John D. Mayer, introduced the world to *emotional intelligence* (EI). According to Mayer and Salovey (1997), emotional intelligence is the ability to perceive emotions, to access and generate emotions so as to assist thought, to understand emotions and emotional knowledge, and to reflectively regulate emotions so as to promote emotional and intellectual growth (p. 1). Mayer and Salovey are the originators of the term and study of emotional intelligence, although Daniel Goleman (1995) is the better known for his best-selling book entitled *Emotional Intelligence: Why It Can Matter More than IQ.*

Many counseling theories have been used to explain human behavior. They include object relations and cognitive, narrative, and behavioral therapy, to name a few. However, a multidisciplinary approach should include the art therapist's primary modality in combination with other assessment tools such as the Bar-On's EQ-I. The Bar-On's EQ-I is a self-report instrument. It was designed as a clinical tool to assess those personal qualities that enable some people to possess better emotional well-being than others (Cherniss, 2000). Assessing for EI has a profound impact on the success and outcome of treatment, but because of lack of knowledge, it is generally omitted when interviewing individuals and families. EI theory and application are important to the field of art therapy. Through the art therapy process, clinicians have access to the client's right-brain graphic narrative (feelings) that activates left-brain verbal narrative or thoughts. Art therapists develop and implement tasks to assist clients who have reached an emotional impasse. If EI is not assessed, clinicians may miss pertinent information related to the client's sense of self, perception of others, and the unconscious material depicted in artwork, resulting in an erroneous diagnosis and therefore treatment.

EI is generally defined as intelligence regarding the emotions, especially in the ability to monitor one's own and others' emotions. Mayer and Salovey established what they call a four-branch theory of EI that includes the following:

1. the capacity to accurately perceive emotions,
2. the capacity to use emotions to facilitate thinking,
3. the capacity to understand emotional meanings, and
4. the capacity to manage emotions.

Families in crisis may be unable to perceive each other's feelings accurately. They may be unable to use emotions and cognition to sustain problem solving. These families are fraught with complex feelings that they are unable to verbalize and believe they may be unable to manage.

Mayer and Salovey (1990) described ways in which people operate in the world, and how family members reach their boiling points, and then become unable to communicate because their words may lead to violence. In conjunction with the research of Mayer and Salovey, Cherniss (2000) purports that EI can help one to "monitor one's own and others' feelings and emotions, to discriminate among them, and to use this information to guide one's thinking and actions" (p. 2).

Although Hein (2005) promotes the EI theory expounded by Mayer and Salovey, he is critical of the two men for omitting ideas he believes are critical. Hein contends that there should be a clear distinction between a person's innate potential and what actually happens to that potential over time. He believes that each child is born with a specific potential for emotional sensitivity, memory, processing, and learning ability and it is these four components that form the core of the child's emotional intelligence. Additionally, Hein posits that this innate intelligence can be either developed or damaged by life experiences, particularly by the emotional lessons taught by early caregivers, i.e., parents, teachers, caregivers, and family during childhood and adolescence. The need to distinguish between EI and innate potential motivated Hein to coin the term EQ (Emotional Quotient), asserting that EQ represents a relative measure of a person's healthy or unhealthy development of his or her innate emotional intelligence. He contends that it is possible for a child to begin life with a high level of innate emotional intelligence, but then learn unhealthy emotional habits from living in a dysfunctional home.

Art Psychotherapy

Today, we read about families in the United States and throughout the world that undergo high levels of trauma, separation, and grief.

Hence, it is possible for individual members and the family systems in general of those families to function with low emotional intelligence, potentially limiting their ability and opportunity to develop in an optimal capacity. The elasticity of "normal families," that is, families with healthy family values, who are empathetic, caring, and compassionate, may be absent in the family schema of distressed families. In less resilient families, counseling may be initiated through the family's interaction with other community agencies, i.e., Children's Protective Services. Distressed families may be guarded and withdrawn until rapport is established between the family and the therapist. Clients have to feel a sense of compassion, trust, empathy, and support in order for them to disclose information that will assist the therapist with further assessment. Often, clients will disclose just enough information to engage in therapy. The art therapist has to be perceptive and be cognizant enough to move the family forward. The therapist's thoughts of "Where do I go from here?" are healthy, and the dilemma should be attended to as soon as possible. Collegial counseling is a good way of working through conflict and indecision. Timing and the method of intervention are critical, particularly if the family is observing the therapist to see if he or she is perspicacious enough to cope with their nonverbal ways of relating. Landgarten (1987) contends that regardless of the type of art intervention, the value of the art task is threefold: the process as a diagnostic, interactional, and rehearsal tool; the contents as a means of portraying unconscious and conscious communication; and the product as lasting evidence of the group's dynamics (p. 5).

I believe the initial assessment should be a collaborative task between the family and therapist. It may involve the therapist talking to the family as a group and/or talking to each family member and then engaging the family in developing the goals of counseling. During the initial session(s), the therapist should assess the emotional intelligence of the family unit and of each individual family member. This is important in order to work with the family at its level of functioning. Emotional intelligence leads to other areas of intelligence that will assist the family in an overall ability to function in a healthier manner. I have found that including EI assessment is an integral part of evaluating the family's mental health.

Families with poor coping strategies may be unable to manage ancillary issues related to emotional intelligence perpetuated by social-emotional crisis. The case study presented in this chapter will demonstrate the efficacy of EI and art therapy in the treatment of an adolescent who suffers from both alexithymia and posttraumatic stress disorder (PTSD), contributory components of the lack of EI. The vignette will demonstrate how the art psychotherapist used the creative process to bypass the client's dissociative impasse due to alexithymia, PTSD, and inadequate EI. Alexithymia is a byproduct of deficient emotional intelligence. In order to understand the correlation between alexithymia and PTSD with respect to the case presentation, it is imperative to have a good understanding of both diagnoses.

Alexithymia: Lacking the Words for Emotions

Alexithymia is a manifestation of a deficit in emotional cognition. People with this problem are generally unaware of their feelings, or don't know what they signify, and hence they rarely talk about their emotions or their emotional preferences. They operate in a very functional manner and rarely use imagination to focus their drives and motivations. Although alexithymia is a clinical construct, it does not constitute a diagnostic illness in its own right. It is a clinical feature associated with a range of medical diagnoses, such as PTSD, anorexia nervosa, and Asperger's syndrome (Alexithymia Information Resource, n.d.). Alexithymia is inextricably linked to EI and PTSD. A comprehensive assessment may involve a paradigm shift in assessment techniques for art therapists. This may include using nonstandard instruments. Collaborative test instruments will assist with understanding the subtle cues in clients' narratives and promote additional probing that may result in families interacting in a healthy self-regulating manner. Understanding the connection between nonverbal communication, EI, alexithymia, and art therapy will be discussed in the case study.

Posttraumatic Stress Disorder (PTSD)

According to the *Diagnostic and Statistical Manual of Mental Disorders IV, TR* (American Psychiatric Association, 2000), "The essential feature of Posttraumatic Stress Disorder is the development of characteristic symptoms following exposure to an extreme traumatic stressor involving direct personal experience of an event that involves actual or threat-

ened death or serious injury, or other threat to one's physical integrity:
or witnessing an event that involves death, injury, or a threat to the
physical integrity of another person:" or learning about such an event
to a close associate (*DSM-IV-TR*, p. 424). For additional information
about PTSD, the reader is referred to the *DSM-IV-TR*.

Another succinct definition of PTSD is outlined by Ocherberg and
Williams, in which the authors document that PTSD used to be associated primarily with the struggles of Vietnam veterans but today this
term is being used to describe the afflictions of a wide variety of trauma
survivors, rape and crime victims, natural catastrophe survivors,
refugees, torture survivors, abused women and children, and in some
cases, survivors of vehicular accidents and technological disasters
(Cited in Matsakis, 1994, p. 16).

A Case Study

CELIA. Celia was a 17-year-old female who was referred by another
therapist. Celia and her two sisters were in therapy because all three
girls had experienced the trauma of being sexually molested by their
stepfather. All three siblings and their mother participated in family
therapy. The referring therapist believed that the sessions would be
more productive if Celia were in therapy with another clinician because
she was "resistive" and would not talk in session. According to the therapist, Celia's behavior seemed to be a major drawback to meeting the
goals of counseling.

Celia came from a family of five children. She was the oldest of the
girls with one older and one younger brother. The family history was
tragic, as both biological parents were drug addicts for many years.
While both parents were inaccessible to the children because of their
addictions, Celia and her sisters were placed in group homes. Her
brothers were able to remain in the custody of family members. Celia
lived in the group home for approximately four years. After the parents
divorced and they completed a drug rehabilitation program, all of the
children were reunited with the mother. Eventually, the mother remar-
ried and thus began the trauma and disingenuous family bond.

The initial session included Celia and her mother. The mother
focused the session on Celia and through her verbal assertions and
metacommunication, made it explicitly clear that counseling was for,

and about, Celia. The family history was virtually gleaned from Celia in individual sessions. After the second session, it was apparent that talk therapy would not be advantageous. It took several weeks and a change in theoretical approach to build a rapport with Celia. Hence, I introduced her to art therapy and the work of Dee Spring (1993), an art psychotherapist specializing in child abuse. Celia enjoyed drawing and was open to doing art.

Celia was encouraged to use her strength in art to retrieve memories in a nonthreatening way, to tell her story symbolically, and to work through her trauma. The healing qualities of art making were explained as a way of people healing their emotional wounds by projecting outwards (on paper, canvas, or other material suitable for imagery) their anxiety, depression, and other feelings. We discussed making art together and how that process could bring out different feelings in each of us. According to Ganim (1999), "Art can produce a vicarious experience for the viewer and elicit an emotional response. . . . Any emotional response will alter an individual's body chemistry, which in turn affects metabolic functioning" (p. 164). When the emotional response is positive and uplifting or cathartic, "it activates the release of healing endorphins into the bloodstream that boost the immune system, reduce or eliminate the stress response, and enhance metabolic functioning, all of which are crucial components in the healing process" (p. 164). Celia became the author of her story by drawing and the art therapist became the witness to her trauma by accepting her pictures unconditionally.

The therapeutic process included an eclectic intervention that integrated art therapy tasks and selective theoretical theories including behavioral and cognitive therapy. The mandala was chosen as the primary drawing intervention that would assist Celia with her art expression and also offer her a safe creative space.

Spring's (1993) treatment of sexual abuse provided a visual and theoretical guide for working with Celia. Spring's treatment is a process consisting of three categories: exploration, relearning, and integration. Spring's procedure includes confronting fears and experiencing the struggle to understand the fears that provoke anxiety. Spring contends that there has to be a structured manner of working with victims of abuse in order to inspire successful outcomes, as evidenced by the following:

> Positive experiences must be allowed to occur so progress can be measured in terms that the victim can understand. Their investigation must be conducted with diligence and commitment. There must be structure,

direction, and understanding. Symbolic metaphor, which has been defined by both the victim and therapist, leads to a method of communicating through phenomenological language and starts the process of getting the unconscious under conscious control, as the invisible is made visible through visible means. (p. 50)

Although weekly collaborations with Celia were productive, it was nonetheless difficult for her to verbalize feelings and to respond emotively to her images. In response to her dilemma, I reasoned that I had to allow Celia time to objectify her art. Wadeson (1980) contends that when feelings or ideas are at first externalized in an object (picture or sculpture) . . . the art object allows the individual, while separating from the feelings, to recognize their existence. If all goes well, the feelings become owned and integrated as a part of the self (p. 10). Unfortunately, this was not the case with Celia. She did not have the vocabulary to express her emotions.

So began the journey of my asking open-ended questions so that Celia could assert whether or not she was having a good or bad day, or if she felt happy or sad. Celia appeared to be displaying a classic example of alexithymia manifested by PTSD. Celia may have been born with at least average intelligence but did not appear to be using her inborn emotional potential to support her emotional intelligence. Hein (2005), as reported earlier, believes that it is possible for a child to begin life with a high level of innate emotional intelligence, but then learn unhealthy emotional habits from living in an unhealthy home. This hypothesis appeared to support Celia's deficit of emotional and verbal expression. Hein's research encouraged me to support Celia further by developing a vocabulary chart from which she could pick words and colors that matched her visual illustrations and that would also assist her in pinpointing emotional triggers.

Alexithymia, posttraumatic stress disorder, and sexual abuse were Celia's primary diagnoses. The vocabulary chart helped Celia to label her PTSD symptoms and metaphors as they appeared in her artwork. It helped to rule out general adolescent behavior versus alexithymia and deprivation in EI and EQ. It also helped Celia to verbalize her feelings about the events in her life. By using the feelings chart, she was able to describe emotions she could only express previously through metacommunication.

Art Process and Recovery

The following drawings illustrate Celia's journey to recovery and the reconstruction of her life. Structured art materials were used to support Celia in giving a voice to her creative expressions. Spring (2001) stresses the iconographic material used in art therapy, heals memories by taking "the emotional charge off of the content" (p. 3).

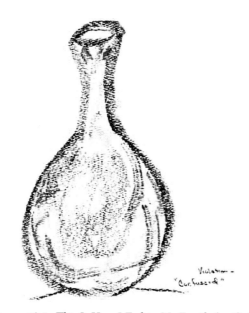

Figure 10.1. *This Is How I Feel in My Family,* by Celia.

Celia's first drawing illustrates the collaborative work of the art therapist and client. Celia used the colors orange, brown, yellow, and black. She stated that the orange represented her anger, and the black represented her. The following client-therapist conversation provides a small window view about the interactive process:

Celia: This is a picture about how I feel in my family. Do you notice anything about the drawing?

Art therapist: Yes, in the inside of the vessel there appears to be figures of some kind.

Celia: The black inside represents me.

The art therapist created the vase image using a broad stroke of purple chalk (client's choice) to encapsulate the client's emotions. The purpose of this collaborative work was two-fold: (1) to establish the symbolic rapport with the client via the art medium, and (2) to provide the client with a symbolic boundary to minimize any possibility of psychic flooding. The art therapist's visceral response to the artwork was that the image appeared to be a baby in utero who was in need of protection. The art therapist's transference evoked sensitivity to the possibility that Celia might be feeling shame, guilt, blame, and self-deprecation . . . hence, the image of one great big ball. Celia stated that the black image represented her; however, as a self-image, the metaphorical representation appears to dissolve in the vase and looks more like what Uhlin calls "blocking out of repression" (cited in Drachnik, 1995). Conversely, it might also represent Celia's feelings of isolation.

The vase drawing was later used to assist Celia's mother in developing empathy and emotional intelligence in relating to her daughter. It also helped the mother to realize that Celia was not resistant to treatment.

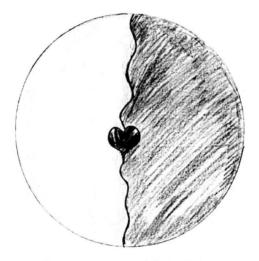

Figure 10.2. *A Mandala*, by Celia.

This mandala illustrates Celia's feelings about her mother. Celia stated that she loved her mother but it was a difficult relationship. The art therapist noted the squiggle line in this picture between Celia and mother that appeared to delineate boundaries between daughter and mother. Celia also displayed ambiguous feelings regarding her mother. The client's affective representation of self was depicted in the color yellow, a warm color. Mother was presented in a light combination of purple and blues, cool colors. It is possible that Celia was projecting an emotional cut-off from mother and she might not have been ready to admit openly that she did not wish to have a relationship with her mother at that time.

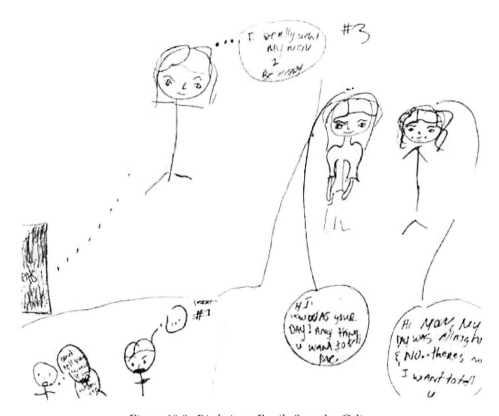

Figure 10.3. *Disclosing a Family Secret,* by Celia.

This picture represents Celia's transition from being a victim. The art process helped to lower her defenses and enable her symbolically to illustrate the coercion and complexities of not disclosing the family secret. In this drawing, Celia compartmentalizes her story, dividing it into three traumatic events: (1) her disturbing relationship with her stepfather, (2) her internal struggle and inability to cope, and (3) her perception of her mother's response. This drawing represents a thera-peutic breakthrough for Celia. Celia had maintained the family secret . . . the sisters disclosed the family secret, leaving Celia feeling isolated.

Secret #1 states, "Don't tell mom, she won't be happy with you." The second stick figure represents Celia with a wide mouth, looking per-plexed.

Secret #2 depicts a door with the word "secret" written on it. Dots lead up to the image of Celia and she states, "I really don't want my mom 2 be unhappy."

Secret #3 shows Celia and mother having a conversation. Mother states, "Hi Celia, how was your day? Anything u want to tell me?" Celia says, "Hi mom, my day was all right & no, there's nothing I want to tell u."

This visual dialogue tells the story of a young girl's trauma and sexu-al abuse. Her artistic expression is regressive. However, as noted by Malchiodi (1990), "Regressive content may also have a psychological basis; the child who is in crisis is restless and anxiety-ridden and may transfer these feelings to art expression" (p. 163). Celia is now able to objectify her artwork and to process the outcome of the product with increased insight and emotional intelligence, as evidenced by her abil-ity to report feeling sad and to connect that cognition to the metaphors in her drawings. Celia's ego strength and resiliency were also evidenced in her ability to compartmentalize her story, thereby reducing psychic flooding. In addition, she was able to "practice" having an empathic relationship with her mother by projecting her feelings outwards, on paper.

Art therapy was a liberating experience for Celia. For Celia, and other children who use art as their expressive language, the following description about color sums up the healing qualities of art:

> Color is the underlying wisdom of your emotional shorthand. It reflects your thoughts, perceptions, and physical sensations but is most often associated with feelings. The colors you use in art, your home, your clothes, and your environment can help you to deepen your understand-ing of your emotional self. (Malchiodi, 2002, p. 151)

Celia is now able to talk with her mother while also finding the words to share her feelings with her sisters. The client-therapist collaboration helped Celia to practice engaging in healthy family dialogues. Celia's sisters have now joined in the art therapy sessions and as a family, they are continuing to break the silence about abuse. This is a family that is showing that they can regroup and function as an open system due to their strength and ability to bounce back.

Family Strength and Resiliency

According to the National Network for Family Resiliency (1995), resilience is the family's ability to cultivate strengths that will allow them to bounce back and meet the challenges of life. Members of families at risk are apt to repeat the errors that have stressed and disorganized their family unless they learn behaviors that provide adaption skills similar to those in resilient families. There has been a proliferation of research on resiliency in children and families since the 1980s. McCubbin, McCubbin, and Thompson (1993) contend that just as individuals that cope well under stress do so with optimism and nurturance, so do families. Opportunities for youth to participate in community life connecting with peers and adults builds resiliency while assisting in changing risk conditions (Silliman, 1998). When we as family clinicians incorporate play and right-hemisphere interventions like art into our sessions, our clients become more resilient, learning naturally how to cope in life crises.

A family schema is a collective set of values, beliefs, and rules. Families that are estranged or vulnerable to risk factors find that in crisis they face hurdles that block their ability to function in a healthy manner. In contrast, in healthy families, resiliency is supported by protective factors like (1) adjustment and (2) adaptation. Adjustment involves the influence of protective factors in facilitating the family's ability and efforts to maintain its integrity and functioning, and to fulfill developmental tasks in the face of risk factors. On the other hand, adaptation can facilitate factors in a family that promote their ability to recover in family crisis situations. It also plays a vital role as a recovery factor in promoting family harmony and balance during a family crisis. Inclusive of the family's ethnic identity, beliefs, and values, the family schema appears to be a valuable resource to guide family behavior and adaptation in the face of family crisis (McCubbin, McCubbin, & Thompson, 1996). Emotional intelligence is an asset to be integrated into family resources. It is pertinent to assessing and understanding the complex makeup of families that require reorganization to develop new ways of functioning.

Summary

This chapter espoused several theories and described areas of family functioning that have to be enhanced in order to facilitate the work with abusive and at-risk families. Families lacking emotional intelligence and emotional potential are prone to disorganization and chaos. This chapter highlighted how art therapy can be a lifeline to both distressed families and resilient families.

Art therapy techniques are highly suited for treatment and intervention with distressed families, especially families that lack emotional intelligence. In fact, it appears to be an optimal way of treating families that are prone to use violence as a characteristic way of functioning. Art therapy is a discipline that can assist these families to learn nonviolent communication and behavior, empathy, and compassion. Additional research is needed to validate these thoughts. Hopefully, future researchers in EI striving to validate the hypothesis that EI is a valued factor in family schema will collaborate with art psychotherapists.

The study of EI is a relatively new phenomenon. Mayer and Salovey (1990), along with other pioneering researchers, have provided clinicians with the tools and theories to contribute to this cutting-edge research. I encourage art therapists to work within the field of EI, leaving a legacy that will include art psychotherapy. Art therapy may be the paintbrush or the marker that provides the missing link in the discovery of how families can reach their highest vitality and emotional intelligence.

References

Alexithymia Information Resource. (n.d.) Retrieved January 20, 2006, from http://www.alexithymia.info

American Psychiatric Association. (1994). *Diagnostic and statistical manual of mental disorders* (4th ed.). Washington, DC: Author.

Berk, L. (1999). *Infants, children, and adolescents.* Needham Heights, MA: Boston: Allyn & Bacon.

Cherniss, C. (2000). *Emotional intelligence: What it is and why it matters.* Retrieved January 15, 2006, from http://www.eiconsortium.org/research/what_is_emotional_intelligence

Drachnik, C. (1995). *Interpreting metaphors in children's drawings.* Burlingame, CA: Abbeygate Press.

Ganim, B. (1999). *Art and healing.* New York: Three Rivers.

Goleman, D. (1995). *Emotional intelligence: Why it can matter more than IQ.* New York: Bantam.

Hein, S. (2005). *Introduction to emotional intelligence.* Retrieved December 12, 2005, from http://eqi.org/history.htm

Landgarten, H. (1987). *Family art psychotherapy: A clinical guide and casebook.* New York: Brunner/Mazel.

Malchiodi, C (1990). *Breaking the silence: Art therapy with children from violent homes.* New York: Brunner/Mazel.

Malchiodi, C. (2002). *The soul's palette.* Boston: Shambhala Publications.

Matsakis, A. (1994). *Post-traumatic stress disorder: A complete guide.* Oakland, CA: Harbinger.

Mayer, J., & Salovey, P. (1990). Emotional intelligence. *Imagination, Cognition, and Personal Intelligence, 9,* 185–211.

Mayer, J. & Salovey, P. (1997). What is emotional intelligence? In P. Salovey & D. Sluyter (Eds). *Emotional Development and Emotional Intelligence: Implications for educators* (pp. 3–31). New York: Basic Books.

McCubbin, H. I., McCubbin, M., & Thompson, A. (1993). Resiliency in families: The role of family schema and appraisal in family adaptation to crisis. In T. H. Brubaker (Ed.), *Family relations: Challenges for the future.* Beverly Hills, CA: Sage.

McCubbin, M. A., McCubbin, H., & Thompson, A. (1996). Family Problem Communication Index. In M. McCubbin & A. Thompson (Eds.), *Family assessment: Resiliency, coping, and adaption inventories for research and practice* (pp. 127–136). Madison, WI: University of Wisconsin.

National Network for Family Resiliency, Children, Youth and Families Network. (1995). *Family resiliency: Building strengths to meet life's challenges.* Ames, Iowa: Iowa State University.

Riley, S. (1994). *Integrative approached to family art therapy.* Chicago: Magnolia Street.

Rosenberg, M. (2003). *Nonviolent communication.* Encinitas, CA: Puddle Dancers.

Shehan, C., & Kammeyer, K. (1996). *Marriage and families: Reflections of a gendered society.* Old Tappan, New Jersey: Prentice Hall.

Silliman, B. (1998, Spring). The resiliency paradigm: A critical tool for practitioners. *Human Development and Family Life Bulletin: A Review of Research and Practice, 4*(1). Retrieved July 24, 2006, from http://hec.osu.edu/famlife/bulletin/volume.4/bull41p.htm

Spring, D. (1993). *Shattered images: Phenomenal logical language of sexual trauma.* Chicago: Magnolia Street.

Wadeson, H. (1980). *Art psychotherapy.* New York: John Wiley & Sons.

Wexler, D. (2004). *When good men behave badly.* Oakland, CA: New Harbinger.

Chapter 11

THE INSTINCTUAL TRAUMA RESPONSE

Linda Gantt and Lou Tinnin

The human trauma response is analogous to the evolutionary survival strategy observed in animals when predators attack them. When trapped, most prey lapse into immobility and analgesia, the freeze state. Human victims respond in the same basic sequence but alterations of consciousness and the subsequent interrupted verbal coding of perception in memory complicate the experience. The usual sequence of responses in humans includes:

1. The **startle:** A predictable alarm response to perceived danger. The trapped rat's startle may include a flurry of instinctual fight/flight action.

2. The **thwarted intention:** In the human, this response comes when the urge to escape or to stop the action is foiled. This is the psychological response that comes with knowing it is too late to do anything to prevent perceived harm. It is usually a brief transition between the startle and the freeze.

3. The **freeze:** This state consists of the instinctual physiological components of immobility, analgesia, and emotional numbing. It has been described variously as paralysis, catatonia, being stunned, or entering a robot-like state.

4. The **altered state of consciousness:** This may manifest as an altered sense of time, depersonalization, or de-realization (not able to stay in reality). It seems to be the human elaboration of the animal freeze, but with a sense of separation from the benumbed body.

5. The **body sensation:** This refers to the nonverbal body experience during the altered state that tends to return later as "body memories" manifested as physical symptoms such as pain, gagging, or hunger.

6. The **state of automatic obedience:** This develops after the freeze state. The person may show a form of obedient catatonia or automaton-like behavior. In some traumatic situations, this state is adaptive. For example, it may permit the heroic facing of danger, as in a combat situation. However, in another situation, such as when the person is a victim of a sexual abuser, automatic obedience may complicate the survivor's understanding of the experience. In retrospect, the victim may feel a sense of complicity and guilt because the victim obeyed the abuser.

7. The final stage is **self-repair:** In this stage, pain returns and the person cares for his or her wounds. This is the time when the person may wash compulsively. It is often followed by grief and anger.

Traumatization

The traumatic freeze state alters consciousness and disrupts verbal coding of experience, resulting in fragmented, traumatic memories that lack narrative closure. The traumatic memory fragments usually contain images of danger and states of alarm. They may intrude into consciousness as flashbacks or into dreams as nightmares.

In addition to these intrusive symptoms, we observe in some children and adults a re-experience of phases of the trauma response that is not like a flashback but is prolonged and, at times, continuous. Every phase of the trauma response may be enacted as a personality trait. For example, there is the perpetually startled, distracted, nervous child who is stuck in the startle state, or the benumbed, spaced-out individual with anesthetic skin who remains in the freeze state. An example of posttraumatic automatic obedience is the "sitting duck" pattern of some victims of childhood sexual abuse. This is characteristic of a person who experienced abuse during his or her childhood. She cannot say no to a perpetrator. The individual with depersonalization disorder may represent a fixed, altered state trauma response, and similarly, the child who seems always to be somatically preoccupied (licking wounds) may represent the self-repair phase of the trauma response. These examples in contrast to Pierre Janet's 1889 (1973) reference to intrusive symptoms as "fixed ideas," suggest rather a fixed state.

Essential Tasks of Treatment

Restorative trauma work requires that the client be able to recall enough of the nonverbal details and images of the traumatic experience to construct a coherent and sequential graphic and verbal narrative of the event. This autobiographical story unites fragmented memories into a beginning, a middle, and an ending, allowing the client and therapist to bring closure to the experience. The instinctual trauma response treatment program is based on a core module of therapeutic procedures designed to accomplish three specific tasks of trauma therapy.

Task 1: Narrative processing: The goal of narrative processing is to bring closure to the traumatic memory. The process is designed to convert memory fragments (including nonverbal images and subjective states of consciousness) into a coherent story that the person avows as past history and no longer reenacts as present experience. The story must include all of the critical elements of the person's instinctual response to the trauma. Children are often eager to tell their stories if they can do it in play or through art. The clinician's job is to provide the means for telling the story and when the story is told, to apply the template of the instinctual trauma response in a way that the child can avow.

Task 2: Resolving dissociation: When a person experiences a freeze state during a trauma, he or she loses the capacity for verbal processing of the experience. Perceptions and sensations are stored without words as nonverbal images and "body" memories. When these images are evoked later by reminders of the trauma, the state of mind that the individual experienced during the trauma may also be aroused and experienced in the flashback. That mental state continues to exist separated from the person's consciousness as a dissociated self-state, frozen in time.

Bringing cognitive closure to the trauma may not resolve the dissociated self-state without specific measures to point out that it is not the person's present life. Tinnin, Bills & Gantt (2002) find that externalized dialogues between the person and the dissociated state promote a rapid integration. A variety of measures are available, but the video dialogue is their preferred procedure.

Task 3: Resolving victim mythology: The assumptive world of the trauma victim is based on the person's sense of being crippled by trauma and trying to survive in a dangerous world. Repair of this mythology usually deals with issues of safety and trust. It is helpful for children to externalize these issues in rituals of play or the creative arts, thereby removing the fear of the unknown. When videotaped and reviewed, this portion of the treatment is found to be conventional and relatively brief (Gantt, L. & Tinnin, L., 2002).

Compulsion to Repeat: Harm to Others, Self-destructiveness, and Revictimization

At least since the late 1890s when Pierre Janet first wrote about the relationship between trauma and memory, it has been widely accepted that what is now called declarative, or explicate, memory is an active and constructive process. What a person remembers depends on existing mental schemata. Once an event or a particular bit of information is integrated into existing mental schemes, it is no longer a separate, immutable entity (van der Kolk & Ducey, 1989). Janet "thought that traumatic memories of traumatic events persist as unassimilated fixed ideas that act as foci for the development of alternate states of consciousness, including dissocialization phenomena, such as fugue states, amnesias, and chronic states of helplessness and depression" (Janet, cited in van der Kolk & Ducey, 1989, p. 139). Janet showed how traumatized individuals become fixated on the trauma; it is as if their personality development has stopped at a certain point and cannot expand any more by the addition or assimilation of new elements. Freud independently came to similar conclusions, as does van der Kolk (van der Kolk & Ducey, 1989), who finds that "many traumatized people expose themselves, seemingly compulsively, to situations reminiscent of the original trauma" (p. 389).

Imagery and Affect

Important in therapy using imagery are the "two aspects of imagery [that influence] the form and function of subjective imagery" (Lusebrink, 1990, p. 124). They are the interaction of imagery and affect and the interrelationship between imagery and resistances.

Imagery and affect are generally processed in the right hemisphere on multiple levels. Because of the close connections between imagery and emotion, all or any part of physiological, schematic, and cognitive information may be amplified, resulting in an information overload. Negative emotions distort images by either transforming them or arresting their flow (Lusebrink, 1990). Resistance may also occur due to a lack of understanding of what is expected, what is the process, and the client's inability to make the "transition from concrete references to symbolic images" (Lusebrink, 1990, p. 125).

Appendix

The following chart created by Gantt and Tinnin (2002) assists the clinician with the sequence of the Trauma Response Model when working with traumatized subjects.

THE INSTINCTUAL TRAUMA RESPONSE

Begin with a safe place drawing and a butterfly hug

Adults	Children
What happening first? Startle–A state of high alert: ready Ready action	Lions and tigers, oh, my.
Thwarted intention: (fight or flight). I am out of fundamental survival mechanisms here.	Oh, no! #$%*
Freeze: Momentary state of immobility or paralysis.	I think I am dead.
Altered state of consciousness: An "out of the ordinary" experience, a dream-like state in which time and perception are changed. May involve an out-of-body experience.	This can't be happening. This must be a dream.
Body sensations: The body remembers sensations of the trauma but cannot code the experience in words.	What's happening to my body!
Automatic obedience: Unthinking compliance with any perpetrator or helper (e.g., medical personnel).	Yes sir! Anything you say, sir!
Self-repair: Sleeping, eating, washing, rocking. Withdrawing to a quiet place.	Boy, I'm glad that's over . . . what a relief! Where's my blankie?

End with a Butterfly hug

Revised with personal permission from Gantt & Tinnin (2002), The Trauma Recovery Institute, W. VA.

References

Gantt, L., & Tinnin, L. (2002). *Trauma recovery: Trauma response lectures.* Notre Dame de Namur University, Belmont, CA. [Videotaped].

Lusebrink, L. (1990). *Imagery and visual expression in therapy.* New York: Plenum.

Janet, P. (1973). L'automatisme psychologique: Essai de psychologie experimentale sur les formes inferieures de l'activite' humaine [Psychological automatism: A test in experimental psychology on the inferior forms of human activity]. Paris: Felix Alcan, (Originally published in 1889).

Tinnin, L., Bills, L., & Gantt, L. (2002). Short-term treatment of simple and complex PTSD. In M. Williams & J. Sommer (Eds.), *Simple and complex posttraumatic stress disorder: Strategies for comprehensive treatment in clinical practice* (pp. 99–119). New York: Haworth Press.

van der Kolk, B., & Ducey, C. (1989). The psychological processing of traumatic experience: Rorschach patterns in PTSD. *Journal of Traumatic Stress, 2.*

Chapter 12

HEALING TRAUMA USING THE INSTINCTUAL TRAUMA RESPONSE MODEL

Doris Arrington and Araea Rachel Cherry

Dedicated to the brave trauma victims around the world who
face their terrors with art.

Introduction

In 2002, Drs. Linda Gantt and Lou Tinnin of the Trauma Recovery Institute (TRI) in West Virginia came to Notre Dame de Namur University (NDNU) as Distinguished Scholars. During the semester they were at the university, they trained students and faculty in their *Instinctual Trauma Response* (ITR) model, a bilateral procedure using both graphic and verbal narrative treatment for individuals who have experienced trauma (see Chapter 11), Both Cherry and I were members of that training. Since that time Cherry and I have treated many clients in our office and trained many others in our classes to use this model. We find it an effective treatment for trauma recovery. This chapter will discuss a few of what we call small traumas (little t) and the Instinctual Trauma Response model. We have found that "small" traumas, disturbing but not life-threatening events differ significantly from person to person (Arrington & Cherry, 2004).

Case Studies

PING HWEI. Our "small trauma" reports begin with Ping Hwei, a 25-year-old woman from Taiwan who had just graduated with a master's degree in marital family therapy and art therapy. Throughout her life she had often felt abandoned by her parents due to the 20 operations she had experienced to repair the cleft palate with which she had been born. Wanting to know more about the ITR and if it would help her feel better, she came to us for both treatment and training.

Ping Hwei's safe place. Each person's sense of a safe place is self-specific. With Ping's many operations to repair her cleft palate, she had learned to go inside and find her own self-soothing experience. Ping Hwei's safe place was visual, hard to describe but easy to draw. When we asked her to draw a place where she felt safe, she quickly identified a circle of soft, cool green surrounded by a warm and sparkling yellow floating in a clear blue sky. To install Ping Hwei's sense of safety, we asked her to give her "self" a butterfly hug* and tap in her safe place.

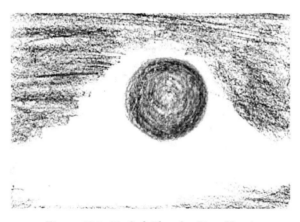

Figure 12.1. *My Safe Place,* by Ping Hwei.

Tapping it in is a simple procedure of alternating hand taps on one side of the arm and then the other. Besides the drawings this also stimulates both sides of the brain.

Next, we asked Ping Hwei to draw what she remembered happening before her traumatic experience. Ping drew what appears to be the operating room with a person she described as herself under the operating room lights. Hooked up to two monitors, she is wrapped in cool, green sheets; yellow lights circle her. The sky blue encompasses the scene. Ping's eyes are wide open; making her look isolated and scared. We asked Ping, since the person in the drawing does not look like a newborn, if she felt this picture represented the first operation or a cul-

* Butterfly hug: Hugging self with both arms and alternately tapping facilitates immediate bilateral integration of the ITR. First introduced in 2003 to Ukrainian counselors by Sr. Mary Duffy and D. Arrington.

mination of all of her operations. She felt that it was a culmination of all of them.

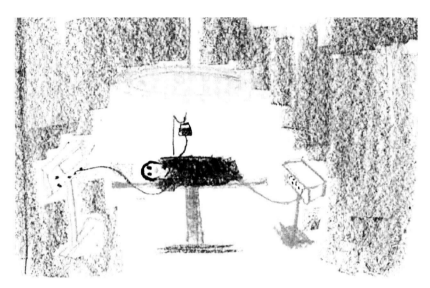

Figure 12.2. *Startle,* by Ping Hwei.

Ping Hwei was then asked to draw what she wanted to do when she realized she was there all wrapped up with no way out. Gantt and Tinnin (2002) refer to this as a *startle,* when the person feels frightened, shocked, or as if he or she is going to die. This picture is a close-up of her face, with her eyes and mouth wide open, and tears running down her face; she is wrapped in a green blanket. She wrote on the picture, "I want out."

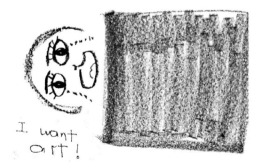

Figure 12.3. *Thwarted Intentions (Flight),* by Ping Hwei.

The next instruction in the Instinctual Trauma Response is to address the person's immediate response. Did she want to run away, stay and fight, or freeze—become immobile? Hwei's next picture is a flight to a momentary state of immobility or an altered state of consciousness. Since the operations had started before she was a month old and had been repeated annually, her survival defenses began as implicit memories rather than explicit ones (see Chapter 2 in this book). Ping Hwei drew a fourth picture of the operating room with her wrapped in the green blanket, eyes and mouth wide open. The sky blue encompasses her in the shape of a box. Providing a tinge of emotion, a magenta color encapsulates the blue. Communication dots connect the blue box with a person with a feminine hairstyle style and arms but no legs encapsulated by both yellow and a green circle. Words above say, "Not me: It's sb [somebody] else! No need to feel pain." The person with the feminine hairstyle stands under a yellow and green encapsulation.

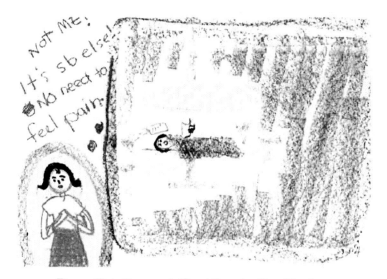

Figure 12.4. *Freeze and Altered State,* by Ping Hwei.

Ping Hwei was asked, who did she think the person with the feminine hairstyle was? She thought and then replied, "It is probably my mother. " Following the ITR model, we ask clients to draw what memories they have of their body sensations. Hwei drew the green box representing the blanket. Again she drew a head but with longer hair, and a furrowed brow. She drew blue lines representing cold around the head. A magenta line also encapsulates this picture. At the bottom she drew a head yelling, "Sb [some body] give her a blanket, she's cold."

Ping Hwei remembers always being cold and her body involuntarily shaking before her operations. She was never quite sure if it was her fear or her body temperature. She always felt alone.

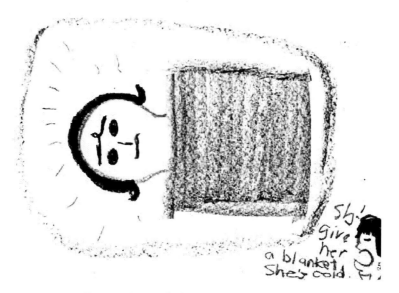

Figure 12.5. *Body Sensations,* by Ping Hwei.

The next ITR question relates to the client's automatic obedience or compliance with anyone in authority. When Ping Hwei was asked if she felt she would do whatever was asked of her in the operating room, she said yes. After the anxiety and prep for the operation, when she was finally in the operating room, she would think, "Oh well, I am here. Let's just get this over with." The picture she drew was of being wrapped in the green blanket, lying on her side, on the operating table. The sky blue is on both sides and underneath the operating table. Above the figure of herself she wrote, "Oh! Well. I'm here. Just get it over with!!!"

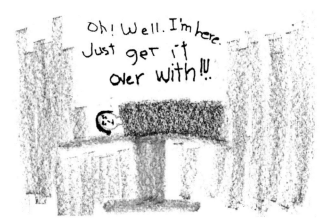

Figure 12.6. *Automatic Obedience,* by Ping Hwei.

The final picture we asked Ping Hwei to draw was how she took care of herself or self-repaired (Figure 12.7). Self-repair is something all humans and animals do. After they have faced some disagreeable event, they eat, rest, talk to a friend, or lick their wounds. For the third time, Ping drew more than one picture on the page. In this picture there are three pictures. The large box shows what appears to be Ping at the bottom of the box with her head on what appears to be a blue pillow and her body under the green blanket. A TV is on a dresser. A small box with perhaps food or gifts is above her head, as are the words "Sleep, rest, read, eat helps to recover soon" written in the sky blue. In the second box, someone is standing next to someone in bed and a box (perhaps a TV) says "On."

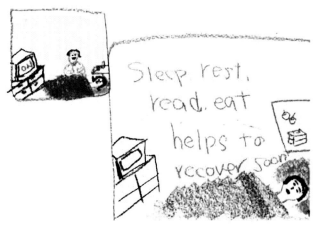

Figure 12.7. *Self-Repair,* by Ping Hwei.

Ping Hwei's graphic narrative was unlocking unconscious material and activating a cycle of transformation (Fosha, 2003, p. 234). When we asked her who she thought the person in the small box was, she said she thought it must have been her mother. Hwei was able to understand that her experience was not of just one operation but a combination of operations over the period of her whole life. She could see that it looked as if she had regressed in the early pictures and aged in the later pictures. She understood and even drew in her pictures that her parents had always been there for her but were not allowed to be in the operating room when she was a patient. She was able to see how her implicit and explicit memories had affected her beliefs. The ITR experience, drawing and talking about each stage, eliminated all of her negative feelings. We asked her to give herself a butterfly hug and bilaterally tap in her good work. Several years later she continued to be at peace, no longer suffering from feelings of abandonment, teaching and using the ITR in her own work as an art therapist in Taiwan.

SARA. The second small trauma case is about Sara, a 21-year-old Canadian volunteer in Kiev, who came to us after returning to the United States, where she was living with her parents because she kept re-experiencing the trauma of witnessing a severely neglected young boy die in a crowded room with people walking and working all around him but no one seeming to pay him any attention.

Sara's safe place. Sara began by drawing her safe place, a green island with one palm tree and two people sitting on the island. There is a golden sun and water on both sides of the island. This is a place Sara and her family visits for rest and recreation. We asked her to give herself a hug and bilaterally tap in this safe place.

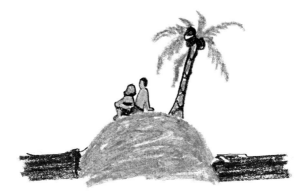

Figure 12.8. *A Safe Place,* by Sara.

Sara' s next picture was drawn in answer to our question, "What happened before the trauma that still concerns you?" Sara told us she was not able to forget one of the first late evenings in the Ukraine when she and her mentor, searching for hungry street children in a still-crowded train station, came upon a small boy, maybe 6 or 7 years old, limp and not moving. Sara drew lines representing the stairs into the train station and a long ledge with two people walking up the stairs. The people represented Sara and her mentor, Tolik.

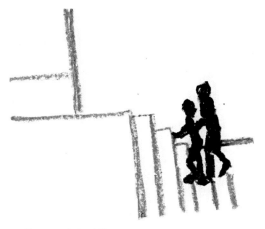

Figure 12.9. *What Happened First,* by Sara.

We asked Sara what startled her that she could not forget. Sara continued, telling us that as the two of them hurried to the small boy, they could tell that he was sinking deeper and deeper into unconsciousness.

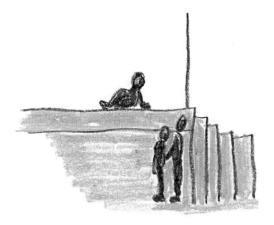

Figure 12.10. *Startled,* by Sara.

Merchants continued to sell and pass by. She reached out for the child, only to know that her fears of him being dead were real. Within moments of her seeing him, he had died in the crowded station with no one around him paying him any attention. As she realized that he was dead and there was nothing that she could do, she suddenly felt sick. Her knees shook, and she felt weak. She believed that her young, healthy body had failed her.

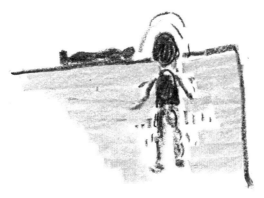

Figure 12.11. *Body Sensations,* by Sara.

She wanted to run away out of the station, out of the evening. She wanted this never to have happened. She thought, "If I have not seen it, it will not have happened. Maybe it didn't happen."

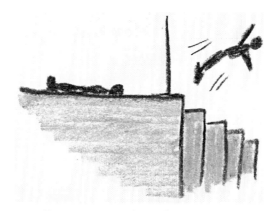

Figure 12.12. *Fight or Flight,* by Sara.

We encouraged Sara to reconnect with her safe space and then to draw how her body felt through this experience. She went over the story once again, saying, "The woman selling flowers next to him just watched him die and then watched Tolik and me like we were crazy because we touched him."

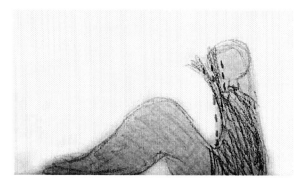

Figure 12.13. *Self Repair,* by Sara.

In response to our asking Sara what she did to feel better, she said she went home and cried and cried. She e-mailed her mom and told her what happened but she felt she had been forever marked by the young boy's death.

Drawing, a right-hemisphere modality naturally connects with right hemisphere experiences and expressions of core emotions. Core emotions unlock unconscious materials, activating a cycle of transformation that helps the patient to feel known, seen, and understood (Fosha, 2003). The Instinctual Trauma Response as discussed by Gantt and Tinnin (2002) taps into core emotional state experiences. Individuals who have been trained in the ITR model assist patients to draw pictures and details of the memories and events that they may need to express, in order to get bad memories out of their systems. The patient will shift from in-the-head thinking to in-the-body sensing and feeling, being in the here and now, embodied in experience. As the patient works through the protocol, he or she will feel more alive, real, and like his or her true self. At this point, we encourage the patients to affirm the experience by giving themselves a butterfly hug, alternately tapping in their experience. Because individuals and their recovery from trauma are individual-specific, operating on their own schedules from idiosyncratic memories, the pictures may fall in a different ITR sequence than the one identified in Chapter 11 (Gantt & Tinnin, 2002). During the ITR process, however, the body of the patient will shift. The patient may take a deep breath and then feel relaxed with energy and vitality. The patient will be able to affirm the self and its transformation. Although for several days after the ITR process the patient may still experience emotional pain, he or she will also feel the healing effect of experiencing positive emotion. They often feel clarity with empathy and compassion toward others. They now understand that the experience is a part of their lives from the past, not their ongoing present (Fosha, 2003).

Postscript. Four years later, Sara has married, completed her B.A., and is currently enrolling in a Ph.D. program where, as a change agent, she will continue her work with children in need.

Additional "Small" Traumas

Additional examples of "small" traumas with which we have used the ITR model follow. However, only selected drawings from the cases are included here.

CHARLIE. Charlie, a 40-year-old unmarried schoolteacher, remembered being 17 years old and coming home with a high school friend for supper. The two teenagers sat down, as Dad, drunk and unsteady, stumbled to the table. Dad raised his voice and slurred his words. As mom placed food on the table, Dad, without provocation, slugged her in the face with his fist. Blood splattered over the dishes on the table and on the food. Charlie and his friend, also covered in blood, retreated to Charlie's room, frozen in fear. Over much of Charlie's adult life, he has retreated in that same state, frozen in fear and depression.

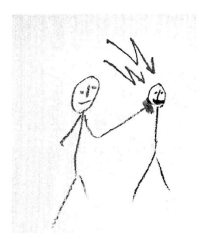

Figure 12.14. *Startled,* by Charlie.

OXANNA. Oxanna, a 35-year-old college teacher, remembers being a 12-year-old, playing with several of her girlfriends in a field near a tunnel that went under a road. A group of rough teenage boys appeared, teasing and taunting the girls with what appeared to be the intent to overpower and harm them. Frightened, the girls picked branches with which to defend themselves, but to no avail. The boys picked larger branches and became more menacing. As if by magic, a truck drove up on the road and the driver stopped to watch the event. The driver motioned to the girls to get in the back. The girls scrambled in the bed of the truck before it drove away.

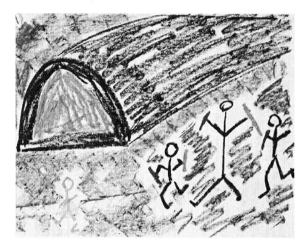

Figure 12.15. *Startled (Fight or Flight),* by Oxanna.

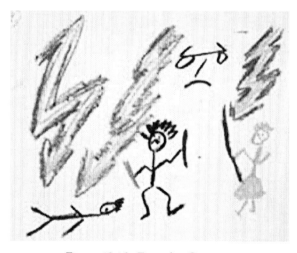

Figure 12.16. *Freeze,* by Oxanna.

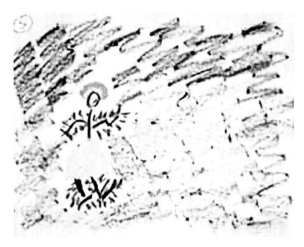

Figure 12.17. *Body Sensations,* by Oxanna.

URI. Uri, a 40-year-old pastor in Eastern Europe, one of seven children, remembers his father's daily beating of someone in the family. More often than not it was his mother. As second from the oldest, he always felt responsible for not protecting his mother. One evening after mother was severely beaten, the father left the home and the mother went to the window in their eleventh-floor apartment. Crying hysterically, she opened the window and was climbing over the ledge when Uri yelled for all of his brothers and sisters to grab her before she fell.

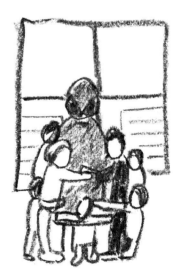

Figure 12.18. *Startle,* by Uri.

He remembers being startled by her choice to jump. For many minutes the children, holding her feet and telling her how much they needed her, kept her from jumping. Uri told his story in a group of about 30 professionals and almost everyone, in sync with his pain, wept when hearing the story.

Conclusion

The human trauma response, according to Tinnin, Bills, & Gantt (2002), is analogous to the evolutionary survival strategy observed in animals attacked by predators. "Human victims respond in the same basic sequence but with more complicated alterations of consciousness and verbal coding of perception" (Gantt & Tinnin, as cited in Arrington & Cherry, 2004, p. 19). Trauma, however, affects not only the victim or victims but also their families. Figley (2000) finds that taking the family into account reduces both victim and family stress. Siegel and Solomon (2003) contend that effective treatment includes right-hemisphere access seen in graphic narrative processing or art processes. Graphic narrative processing unlocks unconscious material, activates feelings, restores memory fragments, and supports verbal narrative processing (telling one's story). Verbal processing converts feelings and memory fragments into a coherent story that the person can avow as past history, preventing it from reenacting as present experience.

Without treatment or with ineffective treatment, traumatic symptoms like absenteeism, truancy, depression, and criminal behavior as well as hospitalization and outpatient medical and mental health treatment can increase. Therefore, it is important that therapists treating trauma patients realize how important trauma treatment is not only for the victim but for the victim's family as well. The trauma therapist, working from a safety model, helps both the victim and her family understand that the victim operates out of a fearful and confusing experience as she works to repair her relationship with self and others (van der Kolk, 2003).

References

Arrington, D., & Cherry, R. (2004). *Trauma and art therapy treatment.* Burlingame, CA: Abbeygate Press.
Gantt, L., & Tinnin, L. (2002). *Art Therapy and Trauma.* Postgraduate course, Notre Dame de Namur University, Belmont, CA [Videotape].

Figley, C. (September 2000). *Clinical Update on Post Traumatic Stress Disorder.* Vol. 2, 5. Washington, DC: American Association of Marriage and Family Therapy.

Fosha, D. (2003). Dyadic regulation and experiential work with emotions and relatedness in trauma and disorganized attachment in healing trauma. In D. Siegel & M. Solomon (Eds.), *Healing trauma: Attachment, mind, body, and brain* (pp. 221–281.). New York: W. W. Norton.

Siegel, D., & Solomon, M. (Eds.). (2003). *Healing trauma: Attachment, mind, body, and brain.* New York: W. W. Norton.

Tinnin, L., Bills, L., & Gantt, L. (2002). Short-term treatment of simple and complex PTSD. In M. Williams & J. Sommer (Eds.) *Simple and complex post traumatic stress disorder: Strategies for comprehensive treatment in clinical practice* (pp. 99–118). New York: Haworth Press.

van der Kolk, B. (2003). *Frontiers of trauma treatment.* Lecture Sponsored by Marin County California Association of Marriage Family Therapist.

Chapter 13

THE POWER OF ART IN HEALING: NANCY'S STORY

Doris Banowsky Arrington and Araea Rachel Cherry

Dedicated to Nancy and to other family members of people
who suffer mental illness and trauma.

In the Beginning

Nancy, suffering from PTSD, had come to us wanting release from the flashbacks and sleep disturbances she had after discovering her husband dead in their backyard. Cherry and I began our process by helping Nancy get comfortable with the office, the area in which she would be working, the art materials available, the video that would be recording the session, the procedure we would be using, and the two of us. Using the Instinctual Trauma Response model (Gantt and Tinnin, 2002), we start by asking all our trauma clients to draw a place where they can relate with safety and security. We want them to have a drawing they can keep in front of them as they work on the trauma that brought them to our office. When they have finished the drawing we asked them to give themselves a butterfly hug installing their sense of safety and security.

"I have had this place for a long, long time," Nancy began: "It is a wonderful garden! The air is clear, the sky is a beautiful blue, and there are lots of trees. I can hear the sound of birds singing and gurgle of the water as it comes out of the fountains. As I approach the garden, I am always a little girl. I always start running toward the garden and as I get closer I get older. Christ always waits for me there and he takes me into his arms. The people I have loved are there in the garden. They all greet me but don't ever engage. The garden is peaceful, restful, and comforting. It is so wonderful that I stay as long as I want." Nancy verbally described her safe place as she drew it, which is rather uncommon. In her first drawing (Figure 13.1, My Safe Place), Cherry and I both noticed that Nancy was drawing haphazardly and disassociating periodically even as she continued to draw and talk. The first session was long and intense, and Nancy felt very tired when she left.

When we reviewed the drawings with her two weeks later, she had no difficulty recounting the incidents in her drawing. There were, however, elements in some of the drawings that were important to the story but she had no recollection of drawing.

After Nancy drew her safe place, we asked her to draw what happened just prior to the startle event (Figure 13.2, Just Prior to the Event). "I came home from teaching school." Because it might make a difference in her memory or her dialogue, we asked Nancy what she was wearing. "What was I wearing that day? Oh, I remember, my red sweater. I have never worn it since. It's in a drawer in a dresser in another room." Nancy became agitated and raised her voice, saying, "I hate that sweater but I have not thrown it away."

One of us normalized this for her by saying, "As we know, people who have been through a terrible traumatic experience often avoid things that remind them of that event." Normalizing is one of the first principles of posttraumatic therapy Ochberg (1993). The idea is to normalize things that are normal (i.e., being afraid or hurt), thus helping the patients see themselves as normal and not feel as if they are weak or mentally ill. Normalization empowers the patient to participate in his or her own recovery process.

Nancy continued. She was filled with the event, the guilt and the shame of it. She kept repeating that she wanted to feel better.

"When I got in the door I called out to Bob like I always did, 'Hi Bob, I am home.' But he didn't answer. He always answered me or appeared. I called again, 'Bob.' My voice raised, *'Bob.'* My stomach immediately went to knots. Bob had been under a great deal of internal stress for the past six months. He had even been hospitalized for depression for several weeks. I did not believe that he was mentally healthy."

Nancy, looking at the picture, said, "This is Bob's car in the garage. No, here," she said with energy, "Here is the first knot. It was when I saw the car, not when he didn't answer me." At this point Nancy drew a small body in the front of the right-hand side of the picture in brown and filled in the stomach area.

Remembering this kind of tiny detail helps people gather together the fragmented pieces of their stories. These memory fragments join the known story elements to form a complete narrative with a beginning, middle, and end. Once the client can avow the story, he or she becomes conscious that the event occurred in the past; it is no longer happening in the present. Now the trauma, as it begins to make sense, can become a story about something that happened to them once. It does not have to be their whole identity.

Nancy began again, "Nothing was out of place from the way I left it in the morning. Not a dish, a plate, a cup, nothing. That was unusual. But then I noticed the sliding glass door was unlocked. I thought to myself, Bob would never leave a door to the house unlocked. He was always getting on me to lock doors. This is when my second knot (Figure 13.3, The small body sensation) came."

"I went back to the front door and called Bob's name. There was no answer. (The third and then the fourth knots came in my stomach.) I went back to the sliding glass door and looked again. I saw nothing. I felt the fifth knot pull tighter. Then I thought, maybe he has just gone for a walk. He would never have done that. He has flat feet and was wearing a brace because his ankle has collapsed. *No, now I remember.* We had gone to get his brace fixed the day before so that he could leave the house. We had even stopped on the way home to buy him some special lunchmeat for his lunch the next day.

"I went back to the glass door and looked out in the yard. There he was down at the end of the yard where Bob had an area that he called his clubhouse. It was a chair he had placed under a lovely little tree that he considered his own private club where he would go to smoke his cigarettes."

We asked Nancy to continue and draw what happened next. "When I first started walking out to Bob it wasn't bad. It looked like he had just fallen asleep. He was kind of . . . just kneeling. I felt like I needed to get to him to see if he was all right."

At this point, Nancy began talking loudly and as quickly as she was drawing. Her processes became very fluid. Her picture changed as her figures changed and she retrieved fragment after fragment of the event that startled her. First, she drew Bob slumped on the ground. Then, as she remembered that he was wearing the blue sweatpants he had always worn since he had gotten sick, she filled in the blue. Next, Nancy drew Bob by his clubhouse; then she begin filling in color, saying, "As I ran toward the clubhouse I saw what looked like a rope around his neck. It didn't register at all. Bob was a terrible, terrible color of green. It was a greenish grey color that I had never seen . . . green grey, weird color, and the rope. It was the rope and the color together that did it.

"Inside I heard this horrible scream beginning in the bottom of my soul, Slowly the scream erupted, drowning out everything else. I couldn't stop it. It was terrible, primal, like something I had never heard before. It was pure pain. I can hear that scream to this day." At this point, tears began running down Nancy's cheeks. She continued to have tears and a runny nose off and on throughout the rest of the session.

Trauma sears memories into the brain. We believe that as Nancy resolved this trauma, the repeated sounding of that scream would abate. The emotional healing process often includes experiencing, avoidance, sensitivity, and self-blame (Ochberg, 1993). These symptoms, set in a context of adaptation and eventual mastery, illustrate a second principle of posttraumatic therapy (PTT): collaboration and empowering (Ochberg, 1993). We checked in with how Nancy felt and when we assessed that she had good ego strength we asked her to continue.

Now Nancy remembered that she had on the red sweater and said, "I still had on that stupid red sweater." At this point Nancy began filling in the red sweater (Figure 13.4, Startle). She said, "The fright was so terrible there was no way I could attend to Bob. It was so terrible I couldn't look at him. But my body moved me. Even if I didn't want to move, it's automatic. Your body just moves you. You don't make any decisions. It just takes over and runs and screams. In the movies when you see someone who has hanged themselves they are hanging down. He wasn't hanging down. There was a stool . . . here." Nancy added the stool to her drawing as she told the story.

Note how Nancy skips around in time, going backward and forward as she recalls more and more about that scene. This is not unusual. The third principle of PTT is the individual principle: Each client has a "unique pathway of posttraumatic adjustment. This is to be anticipated and valued" (Ochberg, 1993, p. 2).

We remind clients to include the little details that come to light in their pictures. We encourage clients to draw their bodies and their body sensations in every picture. We find that this helps prevent unassimilated trauma material from surfacing later as somatic symptoms (body memories), obsessions and compulsions, nightmares and flashbacks, etc. We believe that clients need to include their emotional reactions to the situation as well. For example, "I felt disgusted, I felt angry," etc. If the client says he doesn't know what he felt, we ask him, what does he imagine someone in that situation would feel? If the client is in a group, and I have taught the ITR model to many groups in the Ukraine, Poland, and the United States, I might ask others in the group to add any feelings they might have experienced in similar situations. The client can accept them or not. However, clients will almost always be able to come up with something accurate.

Traumas commonly create emotional, social, and cognitive deficits in a victim's life. To recover from the trauma, it is vital that clients learn to recognize and identify their feelings and start to connect their thoughts and body sensations to those feelings.

As if to cover up all her feelings, Nancy began, in a frenzied state of tears and motion, to add the black color, first making wild black lines, next making long black lines back and forth, and then making short black lines. She made the scene darker and darker.

We sat as silent observers holding the space Nancy needed to retrieve and organize her memories, waiting for her to look up and acknowledge that she needed assistance or was ready to move forward. After a while she stopped and looked up.

We asked Nancy to draw what she did next. Without hesitation, Nancy frenetically drew her sense of derealization, or altered state of consciousness, referring to her self as "another." First she drew at the bottom of the page the lady in a red sweater with hands waving (Figure 13.5, Thwarted Intentions). Then she drew the second lady, saying, "This is another person, a crazy lady. This is another crazy lady! This lady that came running out of this yard is crazy!!! She is crazy with black fright. No one, nobody is there! No one knows the terror!" Nancy's voice was high pitched and expressive. "She is running across the street to the neighbors. She is pounding and pounding on the door. Nobody is coming!" Nancy slowed down. "It seemed as if it took forever, like I was moving in slow motion. Here I am totally alone in the terror. Everything and everyone else is outside this blackness. As this lady runs, she thinks, *someone has to know.* The terrible terror is all over her." Nancy picked up the black oil pastel, peeled it, and colored over everything. Still relating to another, she said, "She almost gets hit by a car."

We want to point this out and normalize this as an excellent example of how people commonly go in and out of the dissociative state during the traumatic event itself.

Nancy, in the thwarted state of flight at this point, said, "It is as if I can't get far enough away. If I can get far enough away it won't be real. It won't have happened. He won't be there. He won't be dead." Note: van der Kolk (2003) supports how our bodies are programmed to move when they feel danger reminds us that during the 9/11 attack people ran for home, believing they would be safe there. Some people ran aimlessly until they wore through the soles of their shoes and their feet bled (van der Kolk, 2003).

Three pictures are interrelated, Figures 13.5, 13.6, and 13.7. Nancy moved back and forth between them, remembering, talking, and adding. She would draw on one a while, lay it down and then move to another, looking and then drawing. We encouraged her many times asking "and then what happened, Nancy? Go with it." Nancy replied, "When you're on automatic you don't see anything. You're just engulfed in the whole event until you don't see anything! Time, distance, and space are distorted." Nancy began drawing multiple figures in blue representing the police with figures of Nancy talking to the figures in blue (Figure 13.6, Altered State of Consciousness). Her lines softened when she drew her daughter encapsulated in the doorway.

"The next thing I knew, it was night. The night happens. You can't stop it; it engulfs you." Nancy used the side of the black crayola to cover the picture. "It is like another person comes into your body and you start thinking weird! I only screamed one scream. A primal scream so loud the next-door neighbor heard it. I have never heard a sound like that from a person before. I ran around the house toward the neighbor across the street. I remember thinking, 'This isn't me running, this is someone else.'" Nancy began to recognize that there was more than one of her in the drawing (Figure 13.7, Altered State of Consciousness–Continued). She had begun drawing her figure on the right-hand side of the paper. We noted the split and normalized it for her, saying, "In this type of situation, dissociation can be a life-saving mechanism. It is one of our earliest defenses. However, what we dissociate from is recorded whole in images, in the nonverbal modules of the brain. That material remains locked in time, often unavailable to the client. If it is to be assimilated, nonverbal information must be retrieved through nonverbal means. Sometimes dissociated traumatic experiences "leak" across dissociative barriers. Old feelings and body sensations may intrude on present-day experiences. Body sensations are the nonverbal body experiences during the altered state. If they are too painful, the person will become numb, as in alexithymia. Otherwise the feelings will return later as body memories or PTSD."

Nancy drew herself in the middle of the right-hand side of the paper and then she used the peeled black crayola to cover her image (Figure 13.7). While Nancy continued to talk, she drew multiple images of herself on the left side of the paper, only one in a red sweater.

"I have no body sensations. I never know when I am hungry or if I am full. I don't know when I have to go to the toilet. I don't feel pain. I don't know what my body needs. I don't connect. I don't confront. I don't take care of myself. That is why there are so many of me. I am numb physically and emotionally. The grey part is the fear of abandonment and not being accepted."

This statement allowed Nancy to see that she had not been shrouded in total nothingness. We watched as she fleshed out the bodies in the picture more closely. Integrating this fragment of dissociated auditory memory made Nancy feel more alive, more present, and more whole. She awakened from the fog. Her graphic and verbal narrative unlocked unconscious material from the trauma. Nancy suddenly declared, looking at Plate 13.5, "There are four of me in this picture, not just one. Finally my neighbor came to the door. I told her, 'I think Bob is dead in the back yard. I think he has taken his own life.' My neighbor had known Bob for 30 years. She couldn't believe it. She went to the phone and called the police. The two of us waited there until the police arrived, then I went back to the house."

Nancy moved in and out of a dissociative state as she drew. She seemed to be collecting memory fragments to add to the story of one time in her life. When we re-presented her story two weeks later, Nancy remembered even more. This time when we asked Nancy how she felt, she began telling us about when she first began dissociating.

"I learned to dissociate very early in life," Nancy said. "Somewhere around third or fourth grade the blackness came in. You're abandoned in this black space. You don't leave here. You shut down everything. You lose the ability to feel anything or know what you even need. You're not alive. You may not be dead, but you are certainly lost! The whole of the pain is contained in this blackness. You are breathing, moving, and existing in that blackness. It covers you and chokes you. It keeps you from living. Don't think about it, don't go there. Just get busy and go on."

Again normalizing this for Nancy, we explained that this sense of numbness is common. However, it sets people up for victimization. One of the essential tasks of trauma treatment is to resolve the victim mythology. Hypervigilance combined with numbness turns people into highly anxious automations. As a result of the graphic narrative process, Nancy connected, making cognitive leaps. She said, "You know, the superwoman suit I have always worn doesn't fit so well. It is worn out and moth-eaten. I am getting too old to do things this way."

Nancy picked up the picture with the police (Plate 13.6) and returned to the trauma, saying, "My mind was racing. I was in a panic. When did this happen? Did Bob eat lunch? I just kept moving, going helter shelter, searching, searching. In my mind I thought he had to have left a note. I was looking for meaning. Moving, searching, looking for something to indicate he was dead. I felt invaded. My town is small and I knew it wasn't possible but it seemed like hundreds of police officers were in the house blocking me from my search. Finally one officer said, 'Ma'am, people who are mentally ill do not leave notes. Alcoholics and people who are depressed leave notes.' But Bob did leave me a note, not the kind that said 'Dear Nancy.' Instead, Bob had arranged all of his affairs. He had put everything in order to take care of me and there were notes with all of his papers telling me where to find the things I would need."

In Figure 13.6 note the chair in the lower right corner of the picture and the telephone in the upper right of the picture. Nancy is holding it. Nancy did not remember drawing the two objects until she recounted the event of calling the children during our second meeting. It is common for people to remember more as they tell the therapist the story. We have the client add these details in the picture at this point. We asked Nancy to draw the body sensations she was having at this time during the event.

Again Nancy used the peeled black crayon to fill in the background. She began drawing a large ice cube on a cart (Figure 13.8, Frozen in Fear). Inside the cube she drew a large golden figure and eight smaller figures. She continued, "I am in an ice cube that is on a wagon. When you want to go anywhere, you just move the ice cube. I stay in this ice cube because guess what, the outside is worse . . . death, suicide, murder, diabetes . . . out here [outside the cube] people say and do terrible things. If you keep your block thick enough you're protected from all that.

"I can breathe alright in that ice cube state. In the blackness, I can't. The black is suffocating. Of the two, I would choose the frozen state. When I am inside, I can decide how I want to feel. My question for me is, do I go in and out of the cube?" Nancy's behavior and art had slowed down. She said, "My grandparents and other people I love are in the garden. Maybe I go in and out of the ice cube to be with them." Note: When we came together two weeks later so that Nancy could re-present her pictures and story, Nancy stated, "I am really in and out of the ice cube. I can't feel much but I can love and be loved. My kids got pretty frozen along with me because they are all inside the ice cube with me. In fact, I have talked about lots of this with my kids. All my kids are married to frozen men, emotionally bankrupt people who have nothing to give.

"The black is a frozen space with no movement. I am not moving at all. It is like death . . . a void. You may be alive but it is a state of death."

The freeze state consists of the instinctual component of immobility, emotional numbing. We have found it is common to go in and out of the freeze state throughout the entire length of the traumatic event. It is difficult to finally get out of it on your own.

Nancy backed up to her picture, Figure 13.3 and said, "I am in blackness. It is absolutely devoid of sound. In the black terror I hear nothing after I heard myself scream until I was aware of the sound of my fists pounding on the door." Next she picked up Figure 13.4, saying, "I was totally alone. Total aloneness . . . it was as if everyone else on this planet had disappeared. The house seemed miles away. There is a black of nothingness. I am totally, totally lost. I think there is certainly not going to be any help in this place. There is no one here to help me."

Note: The experience of total aloneness and isolation is common. Sometimes clients will say they have no memories because they went into a black hole where everything was black. We asked the clients to draw their bodies in that black hole and add body sensations to the drawing. If they protest (which is highly likely), we say something like, "What kinds of things might you have experienced?" When they come up with something, we have them draw that. We want to help our client's bridge from graphic narrative to verbal narrative. We ask them to at least include a head in each drawing. (This is tricky because we don't want clients to make up stories that didn't happen; yet we want to prime their memory pumps, so to speak.) At the Trauma Recovery Institute, every session is filmed, allowing clients to review the sessions with their therapists or to take the tapes home to review them there as well. This offers clients something concrete to which they can relate. In our practice, we film most of our clients as they work through their traumas. We may review the tapes together with the clients rather than send them home.

We asked Nancy to draw how she reacted to the police and her daughter.

The state of automatic obedience (Figure 13.9, Automatic Obedience) develops after the freeze state. In this state, the patient may feel like a sitting duck waiting to be shot.

"I would have done anything anybody asked me to do. You are not yourself at this point. I died. Part of me died with Bob. I am lying face down on the couch. Why am I lying face down? It looks like I am in a coffin with the lid open. This is a twilight area. You need life support when you're like this . . . you want others to feed you, to give you oxygen. You just cannot take care of yourself at a time like this. You can't even get yourself a drink of water." Note: Nancy always drew people from the back, except for three of the little ones in the Frozen in Fear picture, Figure 13.8

Our question to Nancy was how did you take care of yourself? She breathed deeply and drew *Self Repair* (Figure 13.10, Self Repair).

"How did I take care of myself? Well as always, when things get too dark, too crazy, too overwhelming, I just do more. I just work harder. I moved into my many roles. I get into the ice cube and get busy. I take on more and more. I prepared the funeral. I made the poster celebrating his life. I did the eulogy. I got messages. I joined a grief group right away. But you know, people do not want to deal with or talk about suicide. It is a different type of death and people are really unable to deal with it.

When I needed help, my kids rented a little house in the town where they lived so I could be there for the summer. I painted every day. They were the best paintings I have ever done in my life. Bob was healthy at that time and sometimes when he wanted to he would come up and stay for a few days. But I loved being alone. It was the most contented I have ever been. Oh, this is what I need to do. There are too many ghosts in Bob's house. I need to find another place like my tiny house in the country." At the end of our work again we asked Nancy to give herself a butterfly hug and tap in her hard work.

Final Statement

As we prepared for the re-presentation, in which the three of us would again look at the pictures and Rachel and I, as observers, would retell Nancy's story, as in "Once upon a time, there was a lady named Nancy who lived with her husband Bob . . . ," Nancy remarked, "I think when you start drawing there are things that take over and you draw more than you know you are drawing and memory returns. The art did that without me thinking about it."

A Year Later

Nancy called to relay an event. Several weeks earlier, each of her daughters had called to see how she was doing. She felt fine and told them so. One invited her to lunch, another to dinner. She had made plans earlier to take the train to another city to visit a friend and she let them all know that she was busy and couldn't come that day. The morning following her brief trip, her daughters called again to see how her day had been. Only at the end of the phone call did one of them remind her that the day before had been the anniversary of Bob's death. Nancy told me, quite shocked, "I had forgotten it." She told me that prior to the Instinctual Trauma Response treatment, Bob's death was always on her mind. After the ITR treatment she actually forgot for days on end that it had happened. She said she did not believe that she could have gotten through the grief and the shock had she not participated in the ITR. She told me that discovering Bob's suicide is something that she knows she experienced but it no longer lives inside of her, controlling her thoughts or her behavior.

As I talked to Nancy three years later about including her story in this book Nancy told me she lives happily and at peace in the house where Bob died.

Additional information: I had worked with Nancy as a client previously. This is an important piece of information as you need to know how much ego strength your client has before you begin so that you can monitor the timing and questions during the ITR. To gather personal information from a new client may take an additional one or two sessions.

Time involved. We may encourage our regular clients to go through the ITR. However with continuing or new clients we work with them and the ITR until the client feels finished. We allow up to three hours although it may take only one and a half. Because so much is accomplished we believe that this is time well spent. We see an ITR client for the re-presentation and we allow up to two hours. Following the event, continuing and new clients are encouraged to stay in touch with us during the following weeks should they have any thoughts or feelings they do not understand. Clients may have questions earlier but it is not unusual to hear positive reports even a year or two later.

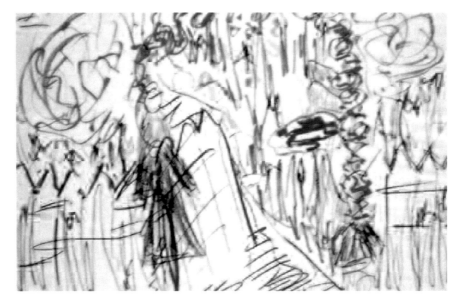

Figure 13.1. My Safe Place.

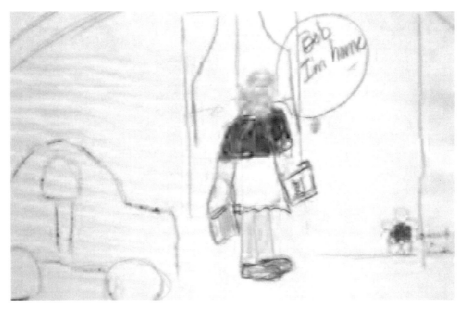

Figure 13.2. Just prior to the event.

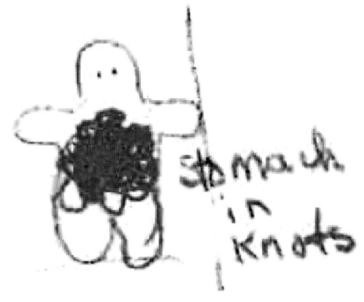

Figure 13.3. The small body sensation.

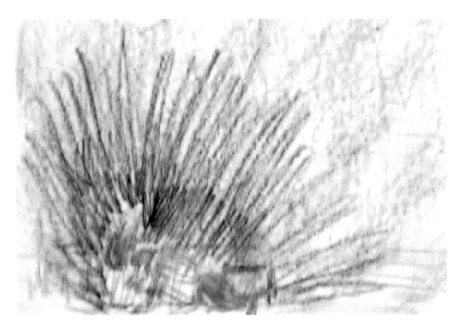

Figure 13.4. Startled.

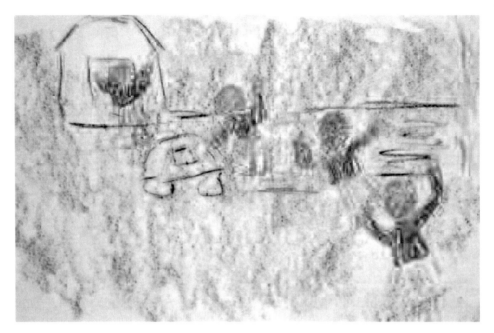

Figure 13.5. Thwarted Intentions.

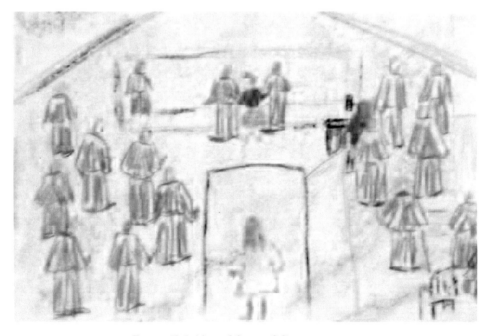

Figure 13.6 Altered State of Consciousness.

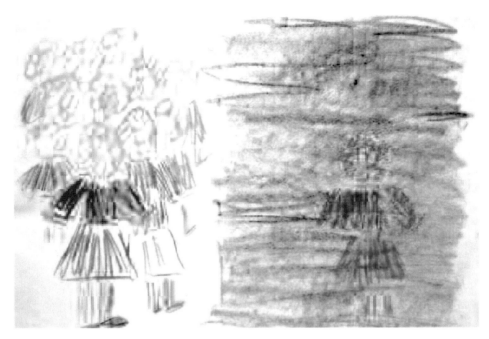

Figure 13.7. Altered State of Conscious-Continued.

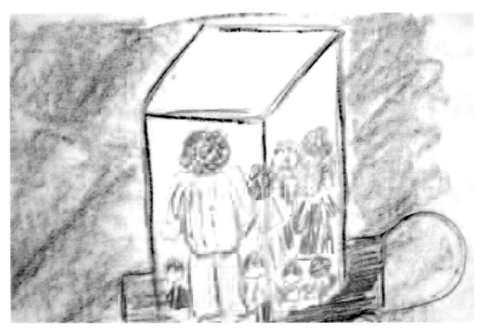

Figure 13.8. Frozen in Fear.

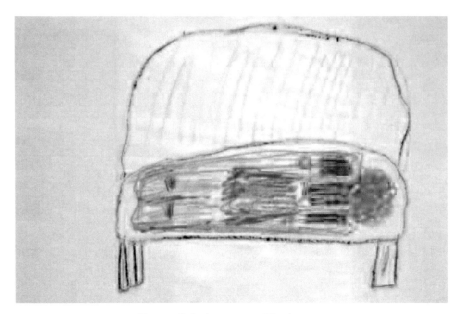

Figure 13.9. Automatic Obedience.

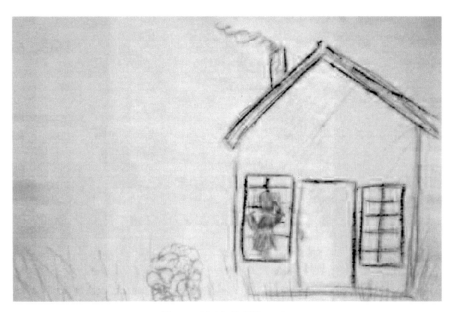

Figure 13.10. Self Repair.

Bibliography

Gantt, L., & Tinnin, L. (2002). *Art Therapy and Trauma*. Postgraduate course, Notre Dame de Namur University, Belmont, CA [Videotape].

Ochberg, F. (1993). Principles of posttraumatic stress. In J. Wilson & B. Raphael (Eds.), *International handbook of traumatic stress syndromes*. New York: Plenum Press.

Tinnin, L., Bills, L., & Gantt, L. (2002). Short-term treatment of simple and complex PTSD. In M. Williams & J. Sommer (Eds.), *Simple and complex post-traumatic stress disorder: Strategies for comprehensive treatment in clinical practice* (pp. 99–118). New York: Haworth Press.

van der Kolk, B, (2003). Posttraumatic stress disorder and the nature of trauma. In M. Solomon & D. Siegel (Eds.), *Healing trauma* (pp. 168–195). New York: W. W. Norton.

van der Kolk, B., McFarlane, A., & Weisath, L. (Eds.). (1996). *Traumatic stress: The effects of overwhelming experience on mind, body, and society*. New York: Guilford Press.

Chapter 14

ART THERAPY IN THE HOSPICE SETTING

Carol Johnson

Dedicated to the memory to my husband, Don Johnson,
whose death led me to this work.

History of Hospice

During the middle ages, a hospice was a place that provided respite for weary travelers. Through the years, hospices have evolved into places where dying patients go for relief of total pain with all of its physical, psychological, social, and spiritual dimensions (Meldrum & Clark, 2000). The modern movement of hospice began in England, in 1967, under the guidance of Dame Cicely Saunders, a physician, nurse, and social worker. The concept quickly spread to Canada, where the term "palliative care" was first used (Saunders, 2005).

Hospices in the United States

The hospice movement in America began in the late 1970s. Today, there are both not-for-profit and for-profit hospices of many kinds in the United States. However, all have the central mission of helping people die with dignity, as free of pain as possible, with their autonomy intact. Hospices provide guidance and support to the patient and the patient's family through the last six months of the patient's life.

For the most part, hospices in the United States care for patients in their own homes. Ninety percent of people surveyed want to die at home, but 70 percent of our population dies in institutions (Hospice of the Valley, Director Sally Adelus, 2005, personal communication at a hospice training lecture). No matter how much people desire to die at home, it is not always possible, so hospices also care for people in hospitals, skilled nursing and residential care facilities, and in-house hospice facilities.

The Hospice Team

A hallmark of all hospice care is the holistic approach envisioned by Saunders. A multidisciplinary team serves the family, providing not only for the medical, palliative care needs of the patient, but for the social, spiritual, emotional and interrelational needs of the family as well. The team is comprised of medical personnel: physicians, nurses, nursing assistants, pharmacists, dieticians, as well as social workers, therapists, chaplains, and a cadre of volunteers. The composition of the teams differs slightly from hospice to hospice, but the multidisciplinary approach is common to all.

At the hospice where I have served for nearly eighteen years, the most important criterion for being a team member, beyond the obvious skills needed, is to have what we have termed the "hospice heart." Many who come to work in hospices do not come for typical career reasons, but to meet a "calling" to serve hospice because they have suffered their own losses to death. Knowing the incredible pain associated with dying and bereavement and the general lack of support found in our culture, those with the hospice heart are highly motivated to help others in their experiences of dying and bereavement.

The Reality of Death

My own hospice heart was seeded by two painful, life-changing events that, within a short period of time, impacted me. The first event occurred in 1981, when acute bacterial endocarditis destroyed my mitral valve. As I lay in a hospital bed for two months with antibiotics dripping in my veins 24 hours a day, I was faced for the first time with my own mortality. I was shocked to find myself in this near-death state, as I had always been the picture of health. I ate sensibly, watched my weight, and jogged three miles several times a week. How could I be this sick and, according to my medical team, possibly on the brink of dying? Though I did not know it, I was experiencing the first of Kubler-Ross's (1969) famous stages of death and dying: shock and denial. In the weeks, months, and years ahead, I would become personally familiar with all of her five stages: denial, anger, bargaining, depression, and acceptance, as well as working through them with countless grieving clients.

One year and twelve days later, after a new valve had been implanted in my heart and I was gratefully alive and beginning to thrive again, my young husband died of a massive heart attack. I was left with four adolescent sons, a still-recovering body, and no local family to assist us. This situation sent me on an urgent search to find grief support for my children and myself. What I found was inadequate and minimally effective.

Birth of a Grief Counselor

With the help of another newly-widowed friend, I started my own support group. I was an art teacher and my newly widowed friend was a journalist. Neither of us had any experience with group support or therapy, so we turned to what we did know and used books as a foundation for our group sessions. Not only did we read and discuss grief books, but we wrote down our experiences and verbally shared our writings as we gathered for our sessions. We encouraged everyone to write, knowing nothing about the therapeutic value of journaling. Our motivation was to capture our grief processes in the hope of collaborating on a book to help other widows. The book never materialized, but the journaling became a foundation stone of our healing. As I had always done during stressful times in my life, I also sketched. Little did I know that the experience was birthing my career as a future grief and art therapist.

Deep in my psyche, an internal transformation was beginning due to the upheaval and reordering of priorities caused by my losses. I had been teaching art in a private school, which did not require a state credential, but now I returned to the university to earn my California art teaching credential. During this period, I instinctively painted a mandala for an art class in response to a directive to paint an internal self-portrait. Having no knowledge of mandalas at the time, I did not understand what I had done, or the significance of it, until several years later. The mandala, an intricate pattern radiating from the center, put me in what I would later discover was the crystallization phase of Joan Kellogg's (1978) Stages of the Great Round. I was definitely living in the present and maturing as an individual, professionally and as a single parent.

Becoming an Art Therapist

Because of my background as an art teacher and what I had seen in children's art through the years, I was drawn to art therapy. Intuitively, I knew that much of what I observed in the art had meaning that I did not understand. Eventually, I was to encounter an art professor, Joy Holm, who held doctorates in both art education and psychology. She encouraged me to take a course she was teaching through a local university. It was entitled "Integration through Art." As I worked with others in the class and began to see patterns and issues that continually arose in our projects, I was astounded by the power of art to help people release and integrate troublesome areas in their lives. It was in this class that my interest in becoming an art therapist was born.

Hospice of the Valley

Training to become an art therapist was one of the richest and most fulfilling pursuits in my life. When I was ready to do my practicum, I knew I had knowledge and personal experience with dying, death, and bereavement that was unique. I asked my physician if he knew of a place where an art therapy trainee would be welcome and could learn to work with dying and bereaved persons. As a member of a local hospice board, he referred me to the director, who was enthusiastic about the use of art therapy in the hospice setting. The director welcomed me as the newest member of her interdisciplinary team.

I became the first of many art therapy trainees at Hospice of the Valley. It has become an agency that knows the value of utilizing art in the healing process of its clients and is always open to innovative ways of integrating art therapy further into its program Today, I direct the Department of Bereavement Services with my assistant director, Bridget Flynn, another art therapist. Some of what will be presented in this chapter will come from the body of work that Bridget and I have developed together.

Grief Counseling vs. Grief Therapy

Hospice work is different from most other therapeutic interventions. Many professionals do not regard it as true clinical work, and hospices themselves call it support counseling. William Worden (2002), who authored the *Tasks of Grief,* which we use as we work with our bereaved clients, states that grief counseling is working with normal grief, whereas grief therapy is working with complicated or prolonged grief. To those of us who work in hospice, it is very fulfilling. We treat our bereaved population by assisting them through one of the most difficult times in life. Almost without exception, those who complete our program leave in a positive frame of mind with new skills to face future losses in their lives.

Art Therapy Begins at Hospice of the Valley

Chris, my first client, was a 12-year-old boy who wanted nothing to do with me, or with grief support. In fact, he told his mother he would run away if she forced him to work with me. Luckily for all three of us, his mother brought him to counseling anyway and soon he and I were busily engaged in art therapy centered on the cancer death of his father.

The Joint Scribble Drawing

The relationship between Chris and I began with a "joint scribble drawing," which has become my standard way of connecting with my young clients. There is something about an adult joining in a child's world of creativity that facilitates and strengthens early bonding. To encourage empowerment, my technique includes letting the child lead at every step of the process. This is important because grieving persons, especially children, feel so little control during the early months of bereavement.

When Chris decided the scribble was complete and had viewed the drawing from all sides, the two main shapes he identified were a hot air balloon and a shape that he identified as a man's tie. He asked me to help him fill in the shapes and instructed me as to which colors to use and where to apply them.

As I watched Chris's hot air balloon come to life with vibrant color, I became aware that the tie shape, located next to the hot air balloon,

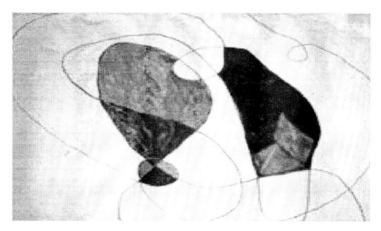

Figure 14.1. *Hot Air Balloon and a Tie.*

looked very much like an Egyptian sarcophagus. This, with a white collar near the top, was eventually painted turquoise. That first day, I did not know the significance of Chris's color choice. I was just aware that Chris used one color, turquoise, in nearly all of his artwork. I was soon to discover it was a connection to the last gift Chris's Dad had given him—a turquoise bicycle that had subsequently been stolen.

Flying Objects

The hot air balloon rising into the sky was the first time I saw a "flying" object in a bereaved child's artwork. It would become a common theme, a wish to "rise above" and "fly away" from the painful circumstances of death. Objects that are commonly drawn include butterflies, airplanes, balloons, kites, rockets, birds, and angels. Some of these symbols have other death significance, of course, but the wish to escape the horror of death is central in the hearts and art of grieving children. In Chris's picture, the combination of the sarcophagus with the hot air balloon was a clear indication of this wish.

Clay Directive Releases Anger

As Chris became more comfortable in my presence, prior to disclosing the loss of the bicycle, it was obvious that his anger was escalating. (Anger is the emotion that most commonly surfaces in grieving adolescent boys.) At the time, we were working in clay, which proved to be the perfect medium for the outward expression of Chris's rage. I asked Chris to make something in clay that represented how he was feeling in relation to his dad's death. While he was in session with me, he repeatedly attempted to come up with an idea. His ideas never felt right to him, and he therefore became increasingly frustrated. He ended up destroying everything he attempted. At the end of our session, an unformed lump of clay remained. I thought the medium was too open-ended for him in his current state, but Chris did not want to give up on the project and asked if he could take the clay home to continue working on the assignment.

A week later, when Chris returned, he had created a large volcano spewing lava. His mother told me that he had spent the early part of the week attempting to create something and then smashing it with a mallet over and over. Finally, when he settled down to work, the volcano formed quickly. Chris was very proud of the clay volcano he had created. When asked how the volcano expressed his feelings about his dad's death, he explained that it was big, like him, and empty inside. The lava that was spilling outside represented Chris's anger that had been allowed to release itself as he worked with the clay. Chris's affect dramatically changed after his experience of working with the clay.

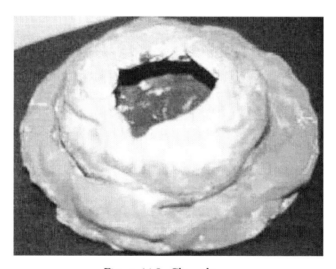

Figure 14.2. *Clay volcano.*

Importance of Linking Objects

When the clay was dry, Chris painted it turquoise with silver lava. This time, when questioned about the color, he explained that turquoise was very special to him because the last gift his dad had given him was the turquoise bicycle. From that point on, turquoise would manifest itself in nearly every art project that Chris did. It became our understanding that his dad was present and Chris felt connected to him every time Chris used turquoise. Chris taught me the importance for grieving people to have connectors (linking objects) to deceased loved ones. In the year that I worked with Chris, the presence or absence of turquoise in his art work would tell me where he was on his path to reconciling to the loss of his dad.

Before- and After-Death Family Portraits

Because Chris was my first bereaved client, I learned much from him and have continued to utilize many of the art interventions and adaptations I used with Chris with other grieving clients. One revealing art directive that we at hospice use in several different ways is to depict life prior to the death and life as it is now. In Chris's case, I had him draw portraits representing the family before and after the death.

In the before-death picture, he drew a normal family with mother, father, Chris, and Chris's brother. Though his dad appeared small and somewhat powerless (he was ill for quite a long time), Chris pictured himself as a child and his mom wore a dress, placing her in the feminine mother role. The two boys were depicted appropriately as smaller than their parents. In the after-death family portrait, the brother was off to one side, while Chris and his mother stood side-by-side. Chris drew himself the same size as his mother, dressed in the same colors as she was wearing. Mother had gone from wearing a dress to wearing pants, much like those Chris was wearing. The roles in the family and Chris's perception of his role in the family—equal to and closest to mom—had changed dramatically. This reflected a common need of grieving children to take care of the remaining parent. If encouraged, the child may see himself as a replacement for the dead mate, resulting in a parentified child role.

During the months we worked together, Chris learned to trust me and I learned to adapt. We used many media and our sessions were fun and productive, though often (understandably) emotionally difficult. As we worked together, I always felt that we were on the path to what thanatologist Alan Wolfelt (2003) calls grief reconciliation.

Chris's last project was a three-dimensional house that he worked on sporadically for several months. In the beginning, the house was only a shell, a shell made of wood and buttressed with mosaic tiles. There was no life in the house, but as the months passed, rooms emerged, then furniture, and finally, as we were ending our time together, Chris made a picture of his dad and placed it in his house on the living room wall. His last touch was putting his own house number next to the front door. Chris and his mom were moving to another state and Chris said that taking his art house with him would mean that he would always have his old house and his old life with him. His house construction served as a linking object to his dad and also clearly illustrated Chris's progress through stages of the grief process.

Art Directives in Grief Work

The art directive "Make a collage of the deceased person showing that person before and after the death" is often given and magazine pictures are provided to make the collage. It is especially effective with adults who are fearful of drawing. Often these collages are amazingly revealing. They show not only changed roles but also the total emotional devastation left in the wake of the loss of a significant other. As familiar as magazine collage is to all art therapists, as well as other therapists who use art without specific training, it is an easy and powerful directive and adapts well in the hospice setting. I often have had clients do series of collages during the year hospice works with them in bereavement. Some of the variations I use in addition to life prior to the death and after the death are: Draw a portrait of the dead person, a portrait of the grieving person (internal and or external), how the world sees the grieving person, how the grieving person sees himself or herself, what the dead person contributed to the life of the griever, what the griever is now missing, how life is now for the griever, and what the griever hopes life will look like in the future. The variations are almost endless and can be adapted to all of the tasks of grief that we use as guidelines to help our grieving clients.

In hospice, even though we would ideally work with patients as well as their survivors, it rarely happens. The reason for this is the severity of illness of our patients. Most are not referred to hospice or choose not to come into hospice until the last few weeks of their lives. By then, they are so critically ill that doing art therapy with them is not a possibility.

Why Use Art Therapy in Hospice?

When asked why one would use art therapy in the hospice setting, I give the following reasons; many are the same reasons art therapy is used in any setting and some are unique to hospice.

1. Art therapy provides a direct line to the unconscious right hemisphere. People, particularly in our death-denying culture, are not in tune with what they are feeling when someone dies. Often, mourners lack the tools and insight to recognize the depth of their grief reactions and are blindsided and overwhelmed by them. Art provides a way for the therapist to help the client identify, name, and process feelings not always accessible through talk therapy alone.

2. Art therapy assists in processing emotions and experiences nonverbally. This appears to be true even when the client never consciously recognizes feelings, and it is particularly true when working with children. One example of this is Star, a 5-year-old girl who was seriously injured in a car accident that killed her 12-year-old brother. (Our hospice also serves community clients whose loved ones did not use hospice. This means we work with a variety of survivors, including survivors of people who died through accidents, heart attacks, suicide, homicide, and other forms of sudden death.)

Star's ability to talk about the accident was limited, but an art project that she did with me shows how she processed and accommodated to what happened to her and her brother.

I gave Star a variety of colored nonhardening clays and a cardboard on which to work. She proceeded to cover the board in green clay and made a black roadway to one side. Next, she created a series of bumps that she called a tunnel. As she worked, she chatted about the road and made lumps of different color clay for cars. She told me that on her road, everyone drove safely and they never had accidents. I could tell that this had to do with what she wished was true, but I didn't know the significance of the tunnel. After the session, she wanted to take her board home intact. She proudly showed it to her mom, who told me later that there was a tunnel just before the accident site. Star clearly was trying to integrate and make acceptable the trauma of the accident

without understanding what she was doing. The art was pivotal in facilitating this process.

Grief Is Encoded into Our Being

In our grief groups, Alexandra Kennedy (2000), who has written several excellent books on grief, is often quoted as noting that grief is
encoded into our very beings. Grief memories, messages, dates, feelings, etc., are present and active in our unconscious even when we are
not aware of them. These are the triggers that create "grief bursts" that
we have in the early years of bereavement, as well as the shifts in mood
that we may have for years afterward. (Art can help to highlight these
triggers, making them accessible for processing!)

An example of this is the common experience of going into a slump
prior to a death anniversary, even years after having ceased to think
consciously of the loss. I experienced this after my husband died. He
died in mid-April. For five successive years, I entered therapy sometime
between the end of March and early April. I remained in therapy for a
couple of months and then was ready to face the world again. Finally,
the fifth year, my therapist observed that I was in a cycle and asked me
what significant events had happened in the spring of the year. When I
began to review my life, I realized that not only had I lost my husband
in April, I had lost my heart valve and three additional family members
during the months of February, March, and April. Once I understood
this cycle, I was better able to cope with my feelings and mood changes
without rushing back to therapy every spring.

3. Art therapy provides containment and control. When a loved
one is ill or dies, no matter how confident and powerful a client felt
prior to the death, he or she is forced into a position of helplessness and
lack of control (Kennedy, 1991). An example of this is a client who
came to us because she had lost her surrogate mother. The client had
been both physically and sexually abused by her birth parents. She had
undergone years of physical and psychological treatment because of
the abuse. As an adult, she developed, for the first time, a love relationship with her surrogate mother that was healthy and unconditional. As
could be expected, the death of this woman plunged my client back
into all of the darkness of her childhood and reduced her to a nearly
primal state.

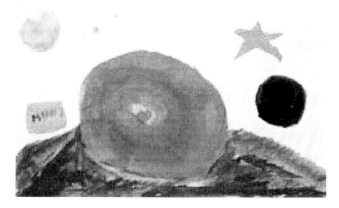

Figure 14.3. *Missing Mom.*

Emotional regression in grief is obvious in this painting, titled *Missing Mom.* The client described herself as the fetal heart in the middle of a blue pillow, her surrogate mother. As she and I worked together, she was able to better contain and control all of the losses in her life through her artwork, which became increasingly healthy. In addition to the art, she also began to put her feelings into words through writing. The combination provided a format for increased control. After a year of our work together, she joined a writing group, finding a new avenue of love and acceptance.

4. Art therapy provides connectors to the deceased. This can take the form of recalling memories in drawings, collages, memory books or boxes, or other art interventions. Connectors are things that will always remind us of the person that died. Physical things are very important transitional objects during the first few months of bereavement, but they also provide concrete proof that the deceased existed for years to come. (This is important because one of the greatest fears of survivors is that their loved one will be forgotten.) Some common connectors are: jewelry, photos, special gifts, wallets, books . . . any items that reminds the bereaved of his or her loved one. I once knew a young widow who carried her husband's slipper around in her robe pocket for months following his death. This was prior to my becoming a widow or a grief therapist and, at the time, I found this attachment very odd. Today, I recognize it as a normal way of coping with her loss. Her husband had been killed suddenly in a plane crash. She needed that concrete attachment object to provide comfort in the midst of her horror.

She needed it, as well, to help her transition into the reality of the death. Other examples of recognized connectors are deceased wives' wedding rings worn on their husbands' little fingers during active bereavement or beyond, favorite items of clothing worn regularly by family members, and perhaps the most contemporary connectors, cremain fragments worn by survivors in crosses, lockets, and bracelets.

5. Art therapy provides a means to ritualize and memorialize the deceased. Grief experts worry about the growing tendency to move away from the historical rituals of death and grief. We no longer hold wakes in our homes, wear black for a year, or prepare our own loved ones for burial. In our death-denying society, we have little opportunity to be exposed to the dead, much less to be educated to recognize the extended pain of bereavement. When death hits, most of us are ill-prepared. We are encouraged to return to "normal" as soon as possible. What well-meaning friends do not understand is that there is no normal for the newly bereaved. It will take months, or even years, before a new normal is forged.

Bereavement Takes Time

A concrete example of the theory that bereavement takes time is the three days of bereavement leave allowed when a primary family member dies. The reality is that it will take months for us to integrate and process the loss. In a recent seminar, Wolfelt (2003), a well-respected thanatologist, stated that any significant loss would minimally take three years to work through. In the case of a losing a child, he says it will take seven years to become reconciled to the loss. These realities do not match up with the expectations of our society, which gives us about six months to adjust to a death. In the average bereavement timetable, six months is about the time when most people finally understand that the dead person is never going to return. It is then that true soul suffering begins. Our hospice staff argues with the *DSM-IV* (1994) terminology that identifies depression past the second month of bereavement as major depression. In our work with thousands of grieving persons over the years, this is often when the normal depression of mourning manifests and the real grief work begins.

Hospice Rituals and Art

To help facilitate ritualization, hospices create sacred spaces and altars on which to place connectors belonging to grieving clients and to the staff who serve the patients. Along with pictures and found objects, we use special art projects made by survivors to remember loved ones. Two examples of these are wood constructions and clay projects made in groups or as we work with individual clients or families. These memorial objects may be used in collective remembrance rituals first and then taken home as permanent memorials to the deceased.

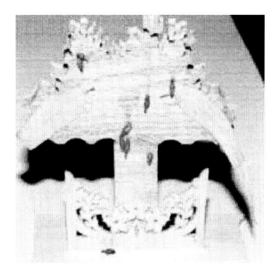

Figure 14.4. *Memorial to mother.*

Figure 14.4 is a memorial sculpture honoring a mother who, as a street person, died under a tree in a park.

The following sculptures were created as part of a family ritual art activity. Family members were asked to make an object in clay that illustrated the special relationship that each of them had with their father, who had died in his early forties of liver cancer. The wife formed a gingerbread-shaped person, cutting a hole out of the center of it. She smoothed the cutout piece into a ball. As she worked, she explained that she felt as if the center of her had been physically ripped from her with her husband's death. (This physical ripping is a common theme in spousal loss.) As the project progressed, she painted one side of the gingerbread person in white and bright rainbow colors, and the other side in black. The colors represented her life of love and joy with her husband prior to his death. The black was where she found herself in bereavement without him. She painted the ball gold and placed it on a blue, undulating pillow shape, which she said represented her husband now. She saw him as beautiful, happy, and free from all pain. He was the golden ball and the blue shape represented eternity.

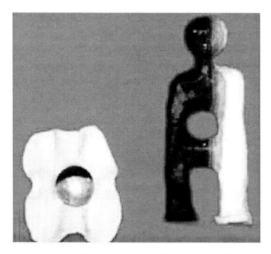

Figure 14.5. *The Helplessness and Emptiness of Widowhood.*

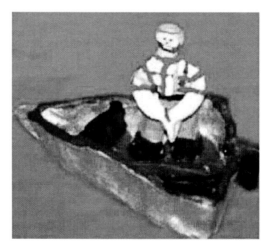

Figure 14.6. *Dad Alone in His Boat.*

The fisherman's boat was the son's tribute to his stepfather. They had spent many happy hours fishing together and as a result had become very close. The son worked very hard at painting in all of the details and wanted this to be a perfect remembrance object for his father. The image of the boat is often connected with death. It is the vehicle the Egyptians used to transport bodies and has long been a symbol of traveling to the next world.

A Case Study: Susan—Trichotillomania Manifested in Grief

Susan, a 12-year-old, who had lost her father was brought to grief counseling by her mother, who was worried because her daughter was pulling out her eyelashes. Her mother thought this behavior was caused by the father's death, which turned out to be only partially the case. This child and her mother were both unable to talk about the pain of the death. Mother was anxious and hovered over her daughter, focusing on the child rather than on her own pain at losing her husband. The child seemed to be carrying the pain for both of them. Both mother and daughter were artistic, so I was eventually able to draw both of them into doing art therapy. It proved a wonderful vehicle for them to learn to name their feelings and begin to communicate more openly about their loss.

Armless clay memorial. Susan was very artistic and chose to depict her father as she remembered him in his last days of life. She sculpted her dad in a chair watching television. Susan had spent many hours watching TV with him as he was dying, and the memories were bittersweet and powerful. As Susan worked, she easily rendered every step of the sculpture until she got to the arms. She placed them in a resting position on the chair, but they never seemed right to her. It took her six sessions to complete the arms, even though they looked fine to me many times in the process. Susan offered no insight as to why she was having such a difficult time with her dad's arms. As I watched her struggle, I sensed it had something to do with the ending of our work together, but more importantly, I knew she wasn't ready to let go of her dad and her grief work around his loss. The arms were significant because the lack of arms and hands clearly illustrated not only her dad's physical helplessness at the end of his life, but also Susan's helplessness in the face of his death. At the last session, Susan finished the arms easily. She was now ready to put her dad and me in a place of memory.

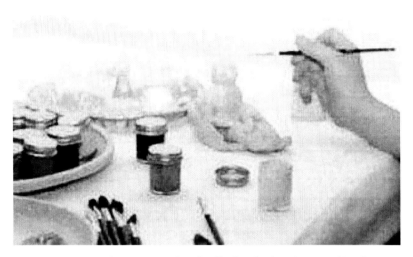

Figure 14.7. Susan paints her finally finished sculpture of Dad.

Susan's trichotillomania slowly improved once she and her mother began to communicate their feelings more clearly to one another. A series of joint sessions beginning with many hours of doing illustrations of grief feelings helped facilitate this process. My methodology for facilitating this was to have them do large pastel drawings illustrating feelings commonly experienced during the grieving process. The drawings completed by the two of them at each session were of one emotion. This provided me with the opportunity to see how they related and communicated. It also helped me identify and normalize their emotional reactions to grief as we discussed what they had drawn and how that related to what each of them was experiencing. My goal had been to provide a vocabulary of grief feelings, enabling them to talk with one another about the death when I was not around to mediate.

6. Art therapy provides a safe way to access, unleash, and discuss feelings. The feeling drawings done by Susan and her mother are perfect examples of safe ways to access, unleash, and discuss feelings using colors, lines, and energy, and they illustrate the importance of the illustrated emotion. *The Tornado of Grief* (Figure 14.8) illustrates the intensity of feelings revealed in artwork, which, as in this case, often surprises the clients.

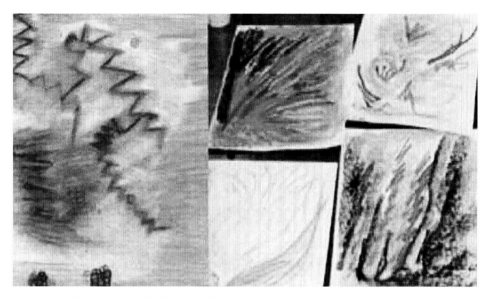

Figure 14.8. *The Tornado of Grief.* Pastel Drawings Release Feelings.

Masks Express Feelings of Grief

Masks (Figures 14.9 and 14.10) are well-known vehicles for accessing and expressing feelings. At Hospice of the Valley, we use everything to make feeling masks, paper plates, clay, ready-made paper maché, and plaster are a few examples.

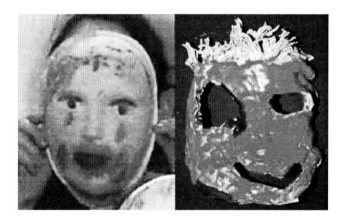

Figure 14.9. Feeling masks.

Preadolescents who were all grieving their fathers made pre-formed masks. A 4-year-old boy whose dad had been killed on a motorcycle did the red clay mask. He called it "happy." The pain he really felt is palpable. The expressions in these masks show the artists' wounding and overwhelming sadness.

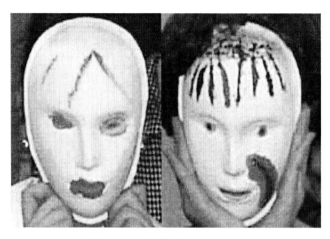

Figure 14.10. Feeling masks.

7. Art therapy provides a tracking tool for documenting progress. Grievers cannot only see their own process and resolution happening, but the group process is visible for all to witness. It is also clear if a client gets "stuck" somewhere in the process. Group members often help people who find themselves in this situation by asking questions that point out the lack of progress or, conversely, encouraging and applauding when they see progress being made by others in the group.

Initially, Sam did not want to participate in a support group. This mandala was done after Sam had bonded with and been encouraged by his fellow art therapy participants. Note the words that show his progress (Figure 14.11).

Art Therapy Combined with Other Modalities

In addition to using art therapy with individuals and families and in art therapy groups, Hospice of the Valley also combines it with other healing therapies. We begin with art therapy and look for other modal-

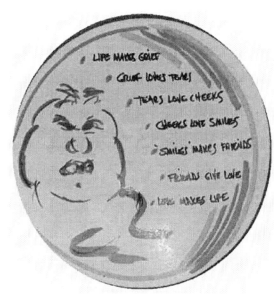

Figure 14.11. *Life,* by Sam.

ities that will help survivors' process their grief in a holistic manner. To date, this effort has included dream work, Tai Chi Chih, journaling, self-acupressure, and storytelling.

The holistic movement at hospice began several years ago when another grief therapist at a hospice convention approached me. He had participated in one of my art therapy workshops and thought it would combine well with his specialty, storytelling. His idea was to suggest an all-day track of "alternate" therapies in the hospice setting for the next convention. The idea was accepted and resulted in an impressive group of different "therapies," including music, sand tray, art, and storytelling, as well as aromatherapy and pet therapy. At the close of the day, a seasoned hospice social worker told me it was the most helpful day he had ever attended because it was experiential from beginning to end. We did a lot of healing work with hospice workers that day. I was fascinated by how powerful it had been to combine art therapy with other modalities and I was determined to try combining it with other therapeutic interventions at our hospice.

By the autumn of 2004, Bridget Flynn had joined our staff as my assistant director. She had been a director at a pain clinic where they combined art therapy and different types of bodywork to help people manage their pain. It was not long before one of our hospice nurses, a

Tai Chi instructor, and Bridget were leading our first art therapy and Tai Chi group. It proved to be a complementary 2-hour pairing. Clients left after the group in a much better space than when they had arrived. This positive change was documented by the use of a pre and post questionnaire each time clients attended group. Measurements were taken in the following areas: physical pain, emotional pain, spiritual connection, and mental distraction. The results were impressive, with changes showing as much as 50 percent consistent improvement in some areas. Our grieving clients' largest areas of improvement were in emotional pain and mental distraction, with spiritual connection also making significant gains.

For our clients, the making of mandalas accesses grief more directly than almost any other art-based intervention. As these feelings are revealed and processed through the art, they are then able to be physically worked through the body by means of Tai Chi. It is a powerful pairing in accessing and processing grief holistically.

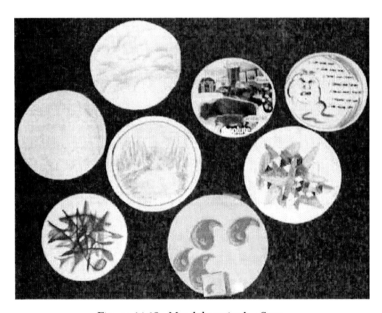

Figure 14.12. *Mandala series,* by Sam.

Sam, a middle-aged man, created a series of mandalas in response to his mother's death. Note the faintness of his early work and the bolder treatments as he became more comfortable with the group. Observe the fragmentation that shows up in so many grief mandalas (Kellogg, 1978). Using art with grieving clients is a powerful tool to help access (and process) the deep angst and pain of losing loved ones to death.

Nearly 20 years ago, only a few hospices were familiar with the advantages of using art therapy with survivors. Today, it is a well-known and sought-after therapeutic modality. Our hospice will continue to search for new ways to use art therapy, alone and in combination with other modalities, in the interest of grieving people and the profession.

References

American Psychiatric Association. (1994). *Diagnostic and statistical manual of mental disorders* (4th ed.). Washington, DC: Author.

Cecily Saunders (2005). *Founder of the hospice movement: Shared letters, 1959–1999.* Oxford, England: Oxford University Press.

Kellogg, J. (1978). *Mandala: Path of beauty.* Towson, MD: Mandala Assessment and Research Institute.

Kennedy, A. (1991). *Losing a parent.* Australia: Harper Collins.

Kennedy, A. (2000). *The infinite thread: Healing relationships beyond loss.* Hillsboro, OR: Beyond Words Publishing.

Kubler-Ross, E. (1969). *On death and dying.* New York: McMillan.

Meldrum, M., & Clark, D. (2000, July/August). Total pain: The work of Cicely Saunders and the hospice movement. *APS Bulletin.* Retrieved July 25, 2006, from http://www.google.com/search?hl=en&q=Meldrum+%26+Clark+Hospice+&btnG=Google+Search

Wolfelt, A. (2003). *Understanding your grief.* Ft. Collins, CO: Companion Press.

Worden, J. (2002). *Grief counseling and grief therapy: A handbook for mental health practitioners* (3rd ed.). New York: Springer.

Chapter 15

RECOVERED MEMORIES: AN ARTS PROGRAM DESIGNED FOR PATIENTS WITH DEMENTIA

Toni Morley and Angel C. Duncan

Dedicated to the wonderful artists who through Memories in the Making create art, laugh, and share their life stories.

Introduction

An estimated 4.5 million Americans have Alzheimer's disease, according to data based on the number of cases detected in an ethically diverse population sample from the 2000 U.S. census. Alzheimer's disease is the most common form of dementia, a brain disorder usually beginning after 65 that affects the elderly person's ability to carry out daily activities. With the aging of the Baby Boomer generation, the projected figures indicate that by 2050, the number of Americans with Alzheimer's could range from 11.3 million to 19 million. One in ten individuals over age 65 gets the disease, and nearly half of those over 85 are affected with it. These figures will have a large effect on our economy in the years to come (Alzheimer's Association, 2006).

Alzheimer's disease can last from two to 20 years and is most commonly broken down into three stages: early, middle, and late. The early stage usually lasts from 2 to 4 years, leading up to and finally including a diagnosis. The symptoms reflecting brain disease include recent memory loss, confusion about formerly known places, getting lost, and lack of spontaneity and initiative. There may be mood or personality changes, or anxiety due to confusion. Often, the affected person exhibits poor decision-making, including trouble handling finances and other daily activities. The middle stage is the longest, lasting from 2 to 10 years. Most notably there is increasing memory loss and confusion, shorter attention span, difficulty recognizing friends and family, repetitive statements, sun-downing (restlessness in the afternoon and evening), perceptual motor problems, and increasing lack of cognitive abilities. The late stage, considered the terminal stage, can last from 1 to 3 years. Persons in this stage can no longer recognize themselves or others. They lose their interest in eating, causing weight loss. They lose their ability to use words, become incontinent, and eventually lose their ability to swallow.

Memories in the Making

While caregivers and families are well served by the National Alzheimer's Association, there are only two known National Alzheimer's Association programs that directly serve the person with dementia. One is for individuals who have recently been diagnosed with the disease, and the other is the Memories in the Making program.

In 1987, a collaborative effort in Orange County, California, between Selly Jenny, an artist and volunteer, and Marilyn Oropeza, an art teacher, resulted in a unique program designed to provide opportunities for individuals with Alzheimer's disease or other dementia to express themselves through art. They called their program Memories in the Making (MIM).

The program uses opaque watercolor materials that provide a way for individuals who have lost the ability to communicate verbally to communicate through creative expression. The success and impact that MIM exhibited in Orange County paved the way for Alzheimer Association chapters nationwide to incorporate the program. Tony Morley was working as a therapist with families of Alzheimer's patients when she was first introduced to MIM. As a lifelong artist, she felt that she had found her fit and immediately began looking for ways to implement the program in Northern California. In 2001, she had this opportunity. The Alzheimer's Association wanted the program to serve diverse communities. The San Francisco Bay Area is a very diverse environment, so she began searching for grants from local and national agencies to provide MIM services to sites in San Francisco and in the two counties on the Peninsula. In the first year, five sites with diverse populations were funded, and since 2001, MIM has expanded each year, with the assistance of the Alzheimer's Association, to include diverse communities in assisted living facilities, nursing homes, and adult day care programs from San Francisco to San Jose.

The multicultural groups include Asians, African Americans, Caucasians, East Indians, Filipinos, and Latinos, as well as volunteers who interpret in languages needed. One of the premises held by the MIM program has been that even if language and culture are different, the art will act as the unifying component. This premise has proven to be true. In MIM settings, artists whose cultures are widely varied sit together, paint, and share their histories and stories through their paintings.

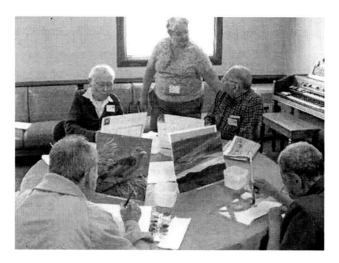

Figure 15.1. Members of the Avenidas group, painting.

The achievements of MIM in the first five sites enabled Morley to hire an assistant director and to take the program to other facilities. Currently, with the assistance of Angel Duncan, they direct and facilitate MIM at 26 residential and day treatment centers throughout the Bay Area.

MIM Goals

The MIM program differs from other arts and crafts programs in its focus on giving dignity and self-esteem back to the artists. It is a fine arts program that encourages self-expression. Coloring books, crayons, cutouts, and glue are not used. The MIM program encourages self-expression that comes from the unconscious and serves as the voice of the unspoken. Goals include increasing self-esteem and sensory stimulation through the creation and sharing of tactile and visual objects.

Therapeutic Benefits

The therapeutic benefits of the MIM program are many. They include productivity, increased self-esteem, and positive affect. There is also more interaction, socialization, a heightened sense of awareness, and an increased sense of belonging among participants in the MIM program. Toshimitsu et al. (cited in Krisztal, Dupart, & Morley, 2003) found that patients with dementia experienced joy in active art therapy and when their artwork received praise by the group leader. Participants and staff find that art is the universal language.

Paint is a fluid medium, and it is believed that this fluidity taps into the right (unconscious) hemisphere of the brain on a preconscious, implicit level, igniting older integrated memory patterns that instantaneously cross bilaterally to the frontal cortex in the left hemisphere, where thought and speech meet (Siegel, 2003). For participants, their internal processes and their interaction with the art therapists assist in memory recollection and their ability to title their pictures. Through the art process and participant interactions with staff and materials, staff members are able to gain insight into the disease process (Kahn-Denis, 1997).

MIM Set-up and Adaptations

The MIM groups of five to ten individuals meet weekly in the activity rooms. Two or three care staff, activity personnel, and often a volunteer or family member assist the art therapist, all acting as "auxiliary egos" for the artists/participants. Communication through painting, fostering connections, and exploring the process of creating are encouraged. Setting up for each group focuses on consideration for vision and mobility impairments. Dark-colored tape is used to define edges of the paper for participants with vision deficits. Brush handles are thickened and weight increased with tape to assist participants in holding them.

On occasion, even hand straps are provided to help the artist/participant hold the brush. Setting up appropriately also means eliminating as many distractions as possible by providing clean and organized areas where participants work. When participants are in wheelchairs, regular chairs are removed from around the table. By offering invitations and reminders, staff assist in gathering participants, often physically wheeling them into group. Due to the short attention spans of the group members, the art therapist helps them start painting as soon as they arrive (Pallet, 2006).

Volunteer, Staff, and Family Assistance

Training staff and volunteers how to use art to work therapeutically with clients is an important part of an art therapist's job. Helping staff learn the importance of an "auxiliary ego," someone that can load and rinse a brush, cue the participant when necessary, and be aware when there is a real need for one-on-one attention, is necessary to the success of the MIM group. Participants in the MIM group have individual needs and different levels of functioning. Knowing these individuals' levels of functioning and abilities, the art therapist can create challenges that keep the participants engaged but not overwhelmed (Pallet, 2006).

Medium Considerations

MIM groups use nontoxic watercolor and high-quality materials that are age-appropriate and foster dignity. Within the group, fluid mediums that lead artists to abstraction are provided, which encourage less focus on getting it "right" that might be the case when using rigid media, like pencils or oil pastels. Staff members have found that three-dimensional media may be mistaken for food and are not appropriate for this population (Pallet, 2006).

Processing of Images

Helping the senior freely associate is an area we find most important when we discuss the painting, reminisce with the artist, and help title the work. This is where the art therapist or the helper can gather the story, connecting the participant's life pieces and memories. This is where assisting the person helps to maintain his or her verbal skills and illuminate his or her mental capacities (Pallet, 2006).

Artists' Stories

As Alzheimer's disease progressively takes away a person's past identity through cognitive decline and lessened abilities, the MIM program supports, appreciates, and encourages the human skills that still remain. MIM is a program about respect and dignity for people who are often isolated and infantilized, yet whose lives have been full of enterprise, travel, love of family, friends, and often art. One of the most significant ways of understanding and appreciating MIM is through the artists' stories. Listening to the stories that accompany the creation of art is a compelling way to help these individuals maintain connection with their families and caregivers.

GORDON. In one of the first groups I ever led, Gordon,[1] a man who had been silenced by the ravaging disease of Alzheimer's, sat down and from a group of pictures on the table selected one of a beautiful tropical fish. For the full 45 minutes of class time, he silently painted his version of the fish. His wife came to pick him up for a doctor's appointment and when she saw what he had painted, she burst into tears. She explained that Gordon had collected tropical fish all of his life. At this point, we all recognized that Gordon's passion was still there, even if he could no longer express it through words. The painting Gordon created once again connected him with his wife and his earlier life. The power of these experiences is very moving. Often whole pieces of lost history come back through the simple act of painting.

JENNY. Jenny, an 85-year-old woman in the middle stages of Alzheimer's disease, suffered from the constant pain of severe spinal stenosis. One day, however, Jenny chose to copy a picture of a pink flower. She was intently painting when I sat down next to her and asked if she had ever seen a flower like that one. I had worked with her for many months, but I had never heard Jenny say more than a word or two. I was astonished when Jenny responded, "Well, my dear, on my thirtieth wedding anniversary, I planned a cruise to Hawaii with my husband and we were on a ship for 7 days. I danced every night and got

---

1. For the sake of confidentiality, all names used in this article have been changed.

dressed up in high heels that matched my dresses, and we had a great time. This flower grows on all of the islands where we stopped." This entire piece of her life's history would have been lost if she had not chosen to paint that faint pink flower.

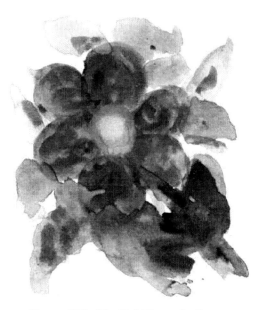

Figure 15.2. *The Pink Flower,* by Jenny.

MARGARET. Margaret, in the late stages of Alzheimer's disease, was invited to come to the group, although we thought she probably would not be suited to it because of the severity of her symptoms (Margaret needed a lot of help simply in selecting and doing). One day, however, with encouragement from the art therapists, Margaret began to paint. She painted blocks of color. The facilitator asked her what her painting reminded her of, and Margaret replied, "I used to make quilts. It looks like a quilt." The facilitator had worked with Margaret for three months, and believed her to be nonverbal, so her ability to communicate and share her past was extraordinary. Margaret continues to attend the MIM group. She currently brings her baby doll and gives the doll painting lessons. Her presence makes a difference and encourages others in the group.

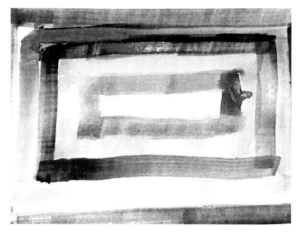

Figure 15.3. *A Quilt,* by Margaret.

DOROTHY. The art produced in the MIM group also serves as a way to bring back memories of past professions. The MIM group members often relive their careers through their art. Dorothy loved coming to the MIM group, but would become frustrated when she tried to replicate pictures of birds, flowers, or landscapes. In her prior life, Dorothy had been a botanist with an interest in fungi, particularly mushrooms. Several images of mushrooms were brought in for Dorothy to replicate, and she was ecstatic. Her face lit up with each mushroom she painted as she proudly announced to the group, "I was a botanist."

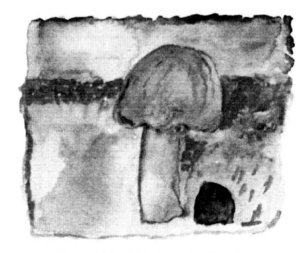

Figure 15.4. *A Mushroom,* by Dorothy.

IRENE. Irene painted a picture of a heart and carefully added squiggles resembling veins. As she painted, Irene kept stating, "I'm a mathematician." When the facilitator inquired about her heart, Irene replied, "It's a heart, a heart with veins that continues to beat. My dream was always to be a doctor. I wanted so much to be a doctor, but I was good in math, and instead I focused on being a mathematician. I'm a mathematician." She gazed at her heart and thoughtfully titled it, *The Beating Heart of a Mathematician.*

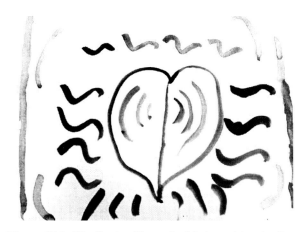

Figure 15.5. *The Beating Heart of a Mathematician,* by Irene.

At the end of the day, the comments most often heard from the Alzheimer's artists include: "That's good!" "I really feel good," "I feel like I did something today." Their faces light up, they stand taller, there is life in their eyes. Once again they have been able to use their own abilities to connect and communicate. It is the process, not the product that is important in this program. Memories in the Making is truly a therapeutic intervention for these clients.

The Memories in the Making program offers a multitude of therapeutic aspects for Alzheimer's patients. The following stories describe how the MIM program has aided those with diagnoses of major depression and Alzheimer's disease.

DAVID. David was in the transition from early to middle stages of Alzheimer's disease, and he was clinically depressed when the facilitator started bringing him to the MIM sessions. David's affect was blunted and he did not engage with others, but he did seem to enjoy participating in the art. In the first few MIM sessions, David painted a farm, and stated that it was his home in the South. The facilitator noticed that David painted only in black. Black may occasionally have a negative connotation, and can be seen as a symbol of grief. Although David did not engage with other class members, he did always thank the facilitators for allowing him to paint. After four weeks and no change in David's choice of media, the facilitator removed the black paint from his watercolor palette and watched to see what other color(s) he might use. David selected the next best thing, brown. Eventually, purple was the only color David used. After about three months, David began using a variety of colors. His mood improved, and he began smiling and engaging more with staff and other class members. He started to talk with the facilitator, who was also from the South, about his life on the farm and how much he loved his childhood. Perhaps their mutual familiarity with Southern culture further enriched their conversation. David, no longer depressed, continued to paint, in color, his farm in Louisiana.

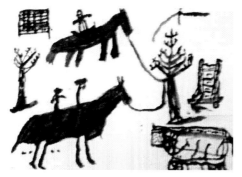
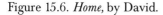

Figure 15.6. *Home,* by David.

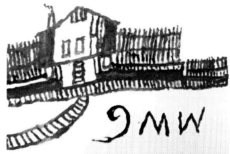

Figure 15.7. *Home,* by David.

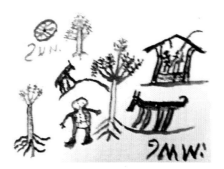

Figure 15.8. *Home,* by David.

ELENA. Elena was a kind woman, always complimenting others and trying to be helpful when the staff was cleaning up. In the MIM class, Elena would focus on her paintings, rarely talking to other group members. In class, she would sit down, swirl colors on her paper, and begin to breathe rapidly, almost in a whirly manner. Elena always included black in her paintings and would announce after each picture, "I like the colors, but not the black. But the black has to be there." Elena's titles for her paintings revealed her inner turmoil. Her entire demeanor would change when she came to the MIM group. But she always left feeling more relaxed, and she would say, "Thank you for letting me come to paint. I feel so much better now."

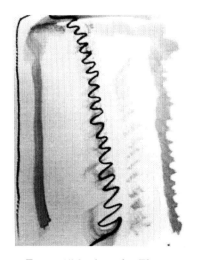

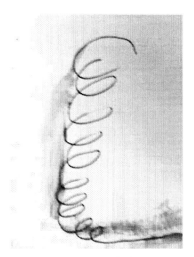

Figure 15.9. *Anger,* by Elena.   Figure 15.10. *Tornado,* by Elena.

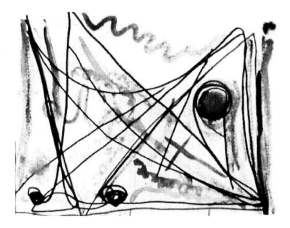

Figure 15.11. *Confusion on the Highway,* by Elena.

Recent Research

Because it is difficult to quantify the therapeutic value of art with inpatients with dementia, there is limited research in this area (Gerdner, 2000). In 2003, Kristal, Dupart, and Morley, in conjunction with the Alzheimer's Association, the Older Adult Family Center, the VA Palo Alto Health Care System, and the Department of Psychiatry and Behavioral Sciences at Stanford University School of Medicine, collaborated on a research study titled "Emotion in Dementia Patients: Effects of a Fine Arts Group on Well-Being." The researchers used direct observation due to the patients' deficiencies in ability to communicate experiences or to respond to traditional psychometric assessments. The instrument used was the Apparent Affect Rating Scale (AARS). Trained raters used the scale to indicate how long a subject displayed each of five emotions over a 5- to 10-minute period. The emotions that they rated were anger, anxiety/fear, sadness, pleasure, and alertness. The Memories in the Making group was compared to the Current Events group. Thirty-five male and female dementia patients between the ages of 65 and 100 years participated in the research project. The qualitative data indicated that in the MIM program, the participants came to life in ways that were seldom seen outside the "art group." Family members reported that after their loved ones had participated in the MIM group, positive emotions carried over to the other areas of life. General observations of the raters were that participants showed more alertness and positive emotion during the MIM group, compared to frequent reports of sleeping, agitation, anxiety, and sadness during the Current Events group.

This study suggests that art therapy provides a more positive outcome for the Alzheimer's population than does a current events discussion group. Art contains the means to enable those with Alzheimer's to reestablish a connection to themselves and to the outside world. As more programs like Memories in the Making are integrated into assisted living curricula, families and health professionals will also accept the importance of using art as a communication component.

While extensive research has been conducted on the effects of music and performing arts on the brain function—further studies in art and brain stimulation need to be conducted to help better understand this disease, and to interrelate how art aids as a fundamental modality for ongoing communicating (Krisztal et al., 2003).

Conclusion

The first annual Memories in the Making conference held in Orange County in July, 2005, provided a way for other Alzheimer's Association chapters and newcomers to learn more about MIM and discuss additional ways to enhance the program. MIM has become more widely acknowledged through recognition by the media, as well as by local and national agencies and gerontology programs, but mostly by word of mouth from the staff of one assisted living Alzheimer's facility to the next as each agency seeks to provide best practices for their residents. MIM, and their art processes and products, provide immediate gratification to patients, families, and staff.

> We were in for such a surprise. We thought that maybe we'd get some response and a little more than what research thought was happening. We were overwhelmed by the gifts that the grateful Alzheimer's patient gave us; they taught us how to deal with them. (MIM staff from Alzheimer's Association of Orange County, personal communication)

Bibliography

Alzheimer's Association. (2006). *Alzheimer's disease fact sheet.* Retrieved January 20, 2006 and July 25, 2006 from http://www.alz.org/Resources/FactSheets/FSAD-Facts.pdf

Alzheimer's Association of Northern California. (2005). *What is Alzheimer's?* Retrieved July 25, 2006 from http://www.alzsf.org/abtalz/abtalz.asp

Alzheimer's Association of Orange County. (2006). *Memories in the making, Art training and round table program.* Retrieved July 25, 2006 from http://www.alzoc.org/home.asp?seltopic1=7&selcategory1=42

Alzheimer's Association. (2006). *View the MIM Scrapbook.* Retrieved January 20, 2006, from http://www.sanalz.org/help_memoriesmaking.htm currently unavailable.

Gerdner, L. (2000). Music, art and recreational therapies in the treatment of behavioral and psychological symptoms of dementia. *International Psychogeriatrics, 12*(1), 359–366.

Hoffmann, D. (Producer). (1995). *Complaints of a dutiful daughter* [Motion picture]. Available from Women Making Movies, 462 Broadway Suite 500WS, New York, NY.

Kahn-Denis, K. (1997). Art therapy with geriatric dementia clients. *Art Therapy: Journal of the American Art Therapy Association 14*(3), 194–199.

Kennedy, R. (2005, October 30). The Pablo Picasso Alzheimer's therapy. *The New York Times,* Section 2, p. 38.

Krisztal, E., Dupart, T., & Morley, T. (2003). Emotion in dementia patients: Effects of a fine arts group on well-being. Unpublished manuscript, Stanford University School of Medicine, Palo Alto, CA.

Macromedia Inc. (1995–2005). Color Wheel Pro: Color theory in action, black. Retrieved September 2, 2005, from http://www.color-wheel-pro.com/color-meaning.html

Pallet, J. (2006). *Art therapy with seniors.* Unpublished paper presented at the Introduction to Clinical Art Therapy Class, Notre Dame de Namur University, Belmont, CA.

Perry-Magniant, R. (2004). *Art therapy with older adults: A Sourceboook.* Springfield, IL: Charles C Thomas.

Rentz, C.A. (May-June 2002). Memories in the Making outcome-based evaluation of an art program for individuals with dementing illnesses. *American Journal of Alzheimer's Disease and Other Dementias, 17*(3), 175–181.

Siegel, D. (2003). An interpersonal neurobiology of psychotherapy: The developing mind and the resolution of trauma. In M. Solomon & D. Siegel (Eds.), *Healing trauma: Attachment, mind, body, and brain* (pp. 1–56). New York: W. W. Norton.

Wadeson, H. (2000). *Art therapy practice: Innovative approaches with diverse populations.* New York: John Wiley & Sons.

Wald, J. (1983, January). Alzheimer's disease and the role of art therapy in its treatment. *Art Therapy: Journal of the American Art Therapy Association, 22*(2), 57–64.

AUTHOR INDEX

SUBJECT INDEX

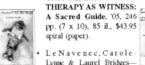

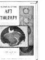

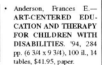

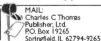